High Praise for *Reflections of a Loving Partner...*

"*Reflections...* is a tender, rich, and colorful memoir of love and loss. For anyone who has ever wrestled with the question of whether it is better to have loved and lost than never to have loved at all, Andrew Martin's memoir shouts a resounding, 'Yes!'"

— *Dr. Ira Byock, Professor, Dartmouth Medical School and Author of* Dying Well *and* The Four Things That Matter Most

"*Reflections...* is both a personal story from a caregiver's perspective and a collection of resources that may support those who find themselves in this challenging role. Everyone who is currently a caregiver, anticipates becoming a caregiver, or unexpectedly becomes a caregiver should own this book."

— *J. Donald Schumacher, President and CEO, National Hospice and Palliative Care Organization*

"The book.... is a valuable reflection for health care providers of... what loving caregivers live in their 24-hour-a-day job of home care. For anyone who has lived the role of caregiver, reading this book will give you solace in sharing this experience that is hard to describe, both in the burdens as well as the joys of serving another."

— *Betty Ferrell, PhD, MA, FAAN, FPCN, Research Scientist, City of Hope National Medical Center; Principal Investigator, ELNEC*

"Andrew Martin has done a beautiful job of sharing his story of struggle and survival.... His description of rituals and ceremonies and his recitation of "remembrance" is clearly articulated through this work. This is a story of hope – taking an unplanned event and turning it into a life's work of great meaning and promise."

— *Pam Malloy, RN, MN, OCN, FPCN, ELNEC Project Director, American Association of Colleges of Nursing (AACN)*

"*[Reflections]...* is poignant, wise, and sweet; a wonderful memorial, allowing me passage through the looking-glass of my profession into unimagined intimacy with a caregiver and his well-loved patient. This book is, among many other things, a recipe for growth at the end of life."

— *Patrick Clary, MD, New Hampshire Palliative Care Service and Author of* Dying for Beginners

"It is tempting to think of AIDS as a disease of the past. While Andrew Martin's experience is retrospective, there is much to learn from his journey and how it continues to influence his life.... Let this book serve as an awakening to our own feelings about caregiving and a reminder to never forget those affected by HIV/AIDS."

— *Gary Gardia, MEd, LCSW, CT*

"Andrew Martin's *Reflections* engages the reader in an intimate journey of love through living, dying, and learning to live and give through it all with deeper intention and care. Andrew's life-lessons gently stir the reader's own substantive reflections about one's eventual dying and ultimately, one's own living today."

— *Joy Berger, DMA, BCC, MT-BC and*
Author of Music of the Soul – Composing Life Out of Loss

"In this intimate memoir, Andrew Martin beams a powerful light into the private worlds of AIDS, hospice training, caregiving, and bereavement. Not only is his story a testament to the transcendent potential of grief but also to the redemptive power of love."

— *Ashley Davis Bush, LCSW*
Transitions and Loss Counselor and Author of Transcending Loss

"Sometimes sentimental, sometimes practical, always brutally honest and moving."

— *Patricia A. Tabloski, PhD, GNP-BC, FGSA, Associate Dean for Graduate Studies,*
William F. Connell School of Nursing at Boston College

"Andrew Martin artfully details the lover's end-of-life experience while simultaneously capturing the capacity of the human spirit. This powerful work denotes human essence, caring, and the magnitude of learning opportunities living and dying both offer when we are open."

— *Lois C. Hamel, PhD, Adult NP,*
Director of Graduate and Online Nursing, Saint Joseph's College of Maine

"All of us wonder if we have 'what it takes' – the strength, kindness, and other gifts necessary to make the best caregivers for our loved ones. This book shares a real-world story of care, loss, and survival. Andrew Martin brings us into his world of caregiving and hope – with loving lessons for life and beyond."

— *Tina Marrelli, MSN, MA, RN, FAAN and Author of the*
Hospice and Palliative Care Handbook *and* Home Health Aide: Guidelines for Care

"*Reflections...* is a gentle guide to self care while companioning a loved one.... The lessons learned from hospice training, woven throughout the memoir, provide valuable insights into... what to do as the end of life approaches.... The author learned the lessons well and graciously shares them with the rest of us."

— *Heather Wilson, PhD, President,*
Weatherbee Resources, Inc., and the Hospice Education Network

"In *Reflections...*, Andrew Martin draws on his personal experience as well as his professional training to provide a thoughtful, useful, and easy-to-read guide to one of the most difficult challenges any of us will ever face."

— *John Rudolph, Journalist/Radio Producer*

"Andrew's story is one that you must read the first time for the joy of the love story, and the second time to share the journey through hospice. The art of storytelling is captured by Andrew as he takes the reader by the hand through each step of.... the intimacies of caring."

— *Betty Brennan, CEO, Beacon Hospice, Inc.*

Reflections
of a Loving
Partner

Caregiving
at the
End of Life

PAUL,
IT'S ALL ABOUT
THE JOURNEY!

by C. Andrew Martin

Quality
of Life
Publishing Co.

Published by:

P.O. Box 112050
Naples, Florida 34108-1929

Toll Free: 1 (877) 513-0099 (in U.S. and Canada)
Phone: (239) 513-9907
Fax: (239) 513-0088

www.QoLpublishing.com

Quality of Life Publishing Co. is an independent publisher
specializing in heartfelt gentle grief support, as well as
books that educate, inspire, and motivate.

Front cover design by Mark May.

ISBN 13: 978-0-9816219-3-7

Library of Congress Control Number: 2010941747

To Lev

"Through the mirror of my mind,
Time after time I see Reflections of you and me,
Reflections of the way life used to be."

"REFLECTIONS"
Words and music by
Brian Holland, Lamont Dozier, and Eddie Holland

Author's Comments

People Change. Diseases Change. Times Change.

People change.

When I wrote this memoir in the mid-to-late 1990s, I was a non-professional caregiver, unprepared for such an unexpected and unwanted role. As part of my grief process following the death of my partner, Gil, I felt an urgent need to document some of the meaningful experiences I encountered as a caregiver; and in this book, I share many of these intimate experiences.

Looking back over the span of time from writing these caregiving vignettes to today, I have earned a nursing degree and worked as a certified hospice and palliative care nurse. I have had the personal mission to create public awareness of end-of-life care issues, not only through my work as a hospice nurse but also as a trained educator for the End-of-Life Nursing Education Consortium (ELNEC) and for the Hospice and Palliative Nurses Association (HPNA). As an adjunct faculty member at the University of New Hampshire, Boston College, and Saint Joseph's College of Maine, I have taught the Death & Dying and Palliative Practicum courses offered through their nursing departments, educating our next generation of professional caregivers. End-of-life care is my passion, and bringing death "out of the closet" is my goal. Yes, people can change through their life experiences.

Diseases change.

The reader of this memoir should also be aware that the face of a specific disease might also change. You will be introduced to a story of love, commitment, and caregiving that took place over a very short period of time, from Gil's diagnosis of HIV/AIDS to his death. That was the rapid trajectory of the disease in the 1990s. Today, with the combination of therapies now available, an AIDS diagnosis carries more hope as a chronically managed disease. With continuing advances in medicine, even the outcome of diseases can change.

Times change.

Although this is a retrospective memoir, some things do not change with time. You may acknowledge changes in both a person and a disease as you read this book, but you will learn that what have not changed with time are the basics of giving care to someone you love.

Caregiving has always been an integral part of the human experience, and some of the basic components of providing compassionate care have not changed with time: active listening, being present, and planning for death. Life Coaching is a popular service that people seek; I propose to offer "End-of-Life Coaching" as an equally valuable learning experience. At the end of this book, I offer exercises relating to select chapters to guide you back to those basics of caregiving. Actively engaging in these exercises may encourage you to have the confidence to become the best caregiver possible, when times and circumstances inevitably shift in your life and you, too, are asked to make that change.

This memoir is the sharing of our true story as a tool to raise awareness of death and dying in today's world. Many of the names and locations have been changed to respect the privacy of those whose lives became intertwined with ours during this caregiving experience. However, it is difficult to completely disguise the identity and actions of certain major players. This memoir was written to illustrate how our saga played out in real life with these major players; it was not written to make judgments about any of their life choices or actions. As it turns out, their choices and actions actually enhanced the universality and reality of our story.

Table of Contents

"STOP! IN THE NAME OF LOVE"

"YOU KEEP ME HANGIN' ON"

"REACH OUT AND TOUCH"

"DO YOU KNOW WHERE YOU'RE GOING TO?"

"LOVE IS HERE AND NOW YOU'RE GONE"

"NOTHING BUT HEARTACHES"

"THE HAPPENING"

"REFLECTIONS"

Introduction

I chose to take care of Gil Victor Ornelas, my life partner, for the final five of his forty-one years. My duties started the day Gil was diagnosed with HIV in the spring of 1991, and they ceased on March 30, 1996.

When I learned of Gil's diagnosis, I searched the bookstores and local library for a guide to prepare me for what may lie ahead. I hoped to find just one book with encouraging words and personal experiences to guide me through each phase of caregiving. I needed answers to the non-medical questions starting to form in my mind:

How will our lives be different dealing with his illness on a daily basis? Will intimacy change with fear of disease? What do we need to do emotionally, spiritually, financially, and legally to be as prepared as possible? Will Gil die at home? Are we ready to take this journey to the end? How will my life go on without Gil? What are grief and mourning, and am I already starting to feel these emotions?

My quest for answers was futile; the books were clinical and impersonal. No single guide satisfied my need for a map that would help chart a course for this excursion into caregiving and care receiving that Gil and I were about to embark upon.

Every caregiving situation is unique, and there are many open roads that lead to the ultimate destination. Every terminal illness requires modifications to the itinerary; there are always unexpected road constructions and detours. Caregiving encompasses more than the physical act of taking care of someone. One must also deal with potential hazards: ethical turns, emotional hills, and unexpected barricades. We encountered many of these when confronted with legal, medical, and financial decisions. Together Gil and I also maneuvered the roadblocks of his family's reactions and subsequent decision to move to another state as they tried to deal emotionally with his disease.

For eighteen months, Gil's outward appearance of good health enabled both of us to deny the virus within. Still searching for that elusive guidebook, I joined a hospice volunteer training workshop as an alternative. This endeavor began to allow open, healthy, and loving discussions about death at home. Lessons learned through hospice training paved the way for Gil's peaceful journey.

The opportunities and choices for caregiving at home – for our family members, partners, and even strangers who become friends – are on the increase. We begin to question: Is this something we have the strength to do? What support will we have if we make this choice? Is this the right direction for us?

Once you say "yes" to caregiving, you encounter many lessons to be learned. The dying person may venture into a slow retreat from the once-shared everyday world and begin to evaluate what is most important during what time is left. I watched Gil slowly lose interest in what he termed "life's small stuff" during the weeks preceding his going into a coma. During the week of the coma, I discovered the magic of communication without words. Once speech and movement involuntarily ended through Gil's body's natural shutdown process, he was able to relay important messages to me through almost undetectable movements: a sudden reaching out of his arms, an almost inaudible whisper of my name, the release of a tear.

"I HEAR A SYMPHONY"

The Diagnosis

The bathroom mirror... Is it the rising steam, fogging the mirror as I shave, which allows the mind mists to clear? Is it the scrutinizing inspection of my exterior that eventually allows the interior to be equally examined? It's been more than two years since Gil's death, yet I vividly replay the events, through the mirror of my mind, every time I see my healthy image reflected.

Gil's Test

"Maybe it's time to get the test." I spoke those frightening words to Gil, referring to the AIDS antibody test.

For many years, every time I had a cold, a swollen gland, a bruise that took too long to heal, or I was just feeling too tired, I questioned the accuracy of my last test results. Any of these symptoms was a sure sign of having been infected with AIDS. Wasn't it?

Beginning in 1985, when the term "gay cancer" was first whispered among the small gay social groups of our New England town of Dover, New Hampshire, I began making routine appointments to be tested twice a year. Even though I was sure this disease was confined to the larger, distant cities of New York, San Francisco, and Miami, I needed the twice-yearly reassurance that there was no virus lurking within.

As a result of the media giving AIDS such prominence, I became a hypochondriac. I needed to know if I was going to become a citizen of the newly forming City of Acronyms – this no-man's land of letter combinations: HTLV-IV, HIV, AIDS, ACV, CMV, AZT, ddI, ddC, MSIR.

It seemed another lifetime, at my annual physical exam, when I asked the doctor to first perform "The Test." Publicity of the epidemic had mounted with actor Rock Hudson's AIDS-related death. Only The Test could squelch my fear of the symptoms I might be experiencing.

The doctor's response surprised me. He suggested I have the test done anonymously at a clinic.

Why at a clinic? I panicked at the thought of executing such an intimate interaction in the company of strangers. He suggested this information should be kept confidential and not a part of my permanent medical files, that I would not want any insurance company to detect from my charts that I was considered at high-risk for contracting this disease. I would not want to be denied medical benefits for what might be lurking in my sexual history. I would not want anyone even to guess at my sexual orientation from a recorded HIV test – negative or positive.

I did not believe such a twentieth-century witch hunt was possible. Nonetheless, it was happening. Single men in their thirties and forties were being denied housing and jobs out of suspicion they were gay. Medical and life insurance policy coverage might be routinely pending until the HIV antibody test results came back from the lab. Panic in the workforce, in health fields, and in neighborhoods was all based on the potential transmission of the virus from these suspect, single, middle-aged men.

But me, at high risk? I again panicked as I tried to remember the names of those I had been intimate with in the past. I calmed myself with thoughts of considering myself at the low end of the risk spectrum. I previously had been in a ten-year relationship, which ended mid-1980, as HIV was gaining prominence. For two years after that, I had dated occasionally and cautiously.

Again, there were the continual nagging thoughts. *Could my first partner of ten years have brought the virus into our home, during a relationship that I had mistakenly thought to be monogamous? Possibly.* I became anxious.

What exactly constituted "safe sex" during subsequent years of dating? Could anyone else have introduced the virus into my world? Another possibility. I almost reached hysteria. Safe-sex guidelines on kissing and other acts were changing on a regular basis.

Did anyone really know the timeframe of the virus's incubation period? Hypochondria. During those years from 1985 to 1987, my semi-annual HIV confirmation test could not come soon enough to dispel my growing panic.

On October 28, 1987, I met Gil Victor Ornelas. My two interim years of casual dating came to an end.

Gil was the most handsome man I had ever met. He was Hispanic-Italian, with dark olive skin; a head of abundant, black curls; dark brown, almond-shaped eyes; and a smile that captured all my five senses. I was in lust. He was gentle and caring, and not like any of the men I had been meeting.

We saw each other only on weekends, alternately driving an hour each way to or from Manchester, New Hampshire, for a six-month period. Because both of us wanted more of each other than the two brief days each week, Gil moved to my hometown of Dover, where we shared an apartment. The first statement of commitment. However, with our different work-shift schedules, we continued to have time together only on weekends, with the added nightly benefit of falling asleep in each other's arms.

After a year of living together, we bought our home: joint property ownership – the ultimate expression of commitment, the closest legal document to a marriage contract between two gay men at that time, before the advent of recognized commitment ceremonies and gay marriage. My life was becoming whole again; I was healing from the end of my first relationship. Gil also felt his life was coming together – and in his case, for the first time.

At the close of the winter of 1991, Gil was out of work for a week. The flu was widespread that winter; the potential of AIDS hovered menacingly in the recesses of my mind. Gil recovered.

But a week later, he was home from work again, tired and running a very high fever. I was anxious.

The following day, when he still had an elevated temperature, I suggested he see my doctor. Now hysteria set in.

Here I was, once again in my doctor's office – this time with Gil – not expecting to hear the same words spoken to me six years earlier. Confirmation of hypochondria.

"Have you had the HIV antibody test recently?" the doctor asked Gil.

"I've never had one," Gil said.

"I suggest you go to a clinic for an anonymous test, just to rule it out." The doctor still promoted anonymous testing. "I'm not saying you have it, but…"

I knew at that very moment, even without confirmation, that Gil was HIV-positive.

Over the past four years, we had never discussed Gil's HIV status. *Did he know and not want to share the information with me? Could it be that he did not know? Did he even care to know one way or the other?* His response – "I've never had one" – answered all these questions.

Did I even want to know Gil's HIV status? Did I wishfully assume he was HIV-negative? Would I want to know if he were HIV-positive? "Yes" to all these questions.

Did I ever once ask Gil, from October 1987 through February 1991, if he had ever had the AIDS test? "No" to the biggest of all questions. HIV status was such a personal issue; but was it too private to ask your partner, when you were involved in a committed relationship? It should not be. He knew that I had been tested routinely before we met.

"Gil, maybe it's time to get the test," I repeated.

"I know, but I guess I don't want to find out." He knew he finally needed to have the test.

"We can go together to the health center where I get tested," I said.

I knew the drill. Anonymous tests were given on Monday nights from 5:30 p.m. to 7:00 p.m. No appointments allowed. You just showed up, were given a number, and sat on a hard chair until summoned by that number – nervously waiting in a room where chances were you knew another "anonymous" person.

Then came the mandatory screening interview. The standard questions never deviated: Are you sexually active? Do you consider yourself at risk for infection? Are your sexual decisions ever impaired by alcohol or drug use? Do you use protection? Do you personally know anyone who is HIV-positive? How would you react if you were to receive a positive test result? After repeated visits, this screening just delayed the result-finding process another fifteen minutes.

Once blood was drawn, the nurse would issue a card with the anonymous identification number. She instructed me to return in two weeks for the result. Two weeks to wait. Results were given only on Tuesday evenings, again from 5:30 to 7:00, no appointments. During two weeks of waiting, the mind plays out every possible scenario of the quality of remaining life once one becomes positive for HIV. Thoughts of tagging personal belongings with the names of those to whom you wish to leave treasures; people to call, perhaps where there has been no contact in years; being more considerate to parents; being more attentive to a life partner.

After two weeks of waiting and wondering, the life-or-death sentence would be pronounced upon the follow-up visit.

But Gil did not know the drill as well as I. "Gil, I'll go with you when you take the test."

"No, I'll do it on my way to work."

The health center was not on his way to work, but the slight detour would add only another half hour to his one-hour commute.

"I'll just be a couple of hours late tomorrow." He worked the second shift, from 3:00 p.m. to 11:00 p.m., at the electric service company as a customer service representative.

"I'll tell my supervisor I have an appointment on my way in."

"Gil, I can meet you at the health center on my way home from work." I remember how intimidating it had been for me to go for my first test, so many years ago.

"No. I need to do this one by myself." His tone showed he meant it.

———

Gil went for the test, and we began the two weeks of waiting. The test became a taboo topic of conversation between us. Life crawled along. Scenarios of Gil living with AIDS played in my head. Were they playing in his? I tried not to get worked up prematurely. Contrary to what I believed, I repeatedly reminded myself that his result could be negative, just as mine had been for years.

"I'm going in tonight." Two weeks had passed. Gil did not seem outwardly nervous.

"May I come along with you?"

"No, you don't have to go just to hold my hand." He wanted to sound brave.

"Okay, Gil. Whatever works for you." I wanted to be there with him, and yet I did not. I could not bear to hear aloud those words, "Your test came back positive for HIV."

———

Our work schedules of opposing shifts allowed us only weekends with shared time; and our solution was to communicate daily by phone each night at 7:30, while Gil was on his dinner break.

It was 7:45 that night, and I had not yet heard from him. I scanned the newspaper to see if there might be a distracting movie on television. *Longtime Companion.* How appropriate, an AIDS movie. I had not yet seen it. As I debated with myself whether to watch it, the telephone rang.

"Hello," I said, expecting to hear Gil's voice.

"I'm positive." No greeting from him other than the death sentence.

"What did you say?" I had heard what he said, but I did not want to believe it.

"You heard me." Silence. "I won't say it again, ever." Deathly silence. "Someone here might be listening."

"Gil, come home, now." I needed to hold him, comfort him, make his hurt go away. I wanted him to make my hurt go away – although I knew it never would go away for either of us.

"It's busy and we're understaffed. I have to stay here." Silence. "I'll see you at midnight." Deathly silence. "Try to wait up for me."

"Gil, I..." I had no more words.

"We'll talk later. Bye."

Silence at the other end of the telephone line. I could not complete the action to hang up the receiver. I held it close to my ear as if it were a seashell, expecting and hoping to hear the ocean's roar.

I could hear nothing but *"I'm positive."* How could he say those words so clinically over the telephone? Why didn't he wait until he came home that night to tell me in person?

I knew he had to share it with me as soon as he could. It was lifting some of the burden of death from his shoulders. My mind had played and replayed this verdict every day – and all day – for two weeks.

Gil and Andrew, welcome to the City of Acronyms. I knew the numbered street signs even though I had not yet traveled there.

Gil would be home in four hours. I could watch *Longtime Companion*. As I was immersed in the film, centered on AIDS and death, I placed Gil and myself in the roles of the leading characters.

What about me? It had been six months since my last test. Lately, I had been going only yearly. Was I also HIV-positive? We had not been practicing safe sex. Regardless of my status – negative or positive – our world had changed. *Longtime Companion* ended, without my realizing it. The next sound I heard was metal touching metal, Gil's key opening the front door lock.

"I'm home." He did not look to me as if he were dying.

"Gil, I..." Again, no words.

We hugged for an eternity until he released my hold on him. "You need to get tested again," he declared.

"What difference would it make?" I asked, although I suspected knowing my status would make a huge difference. I just wanted our conversation that night to focus on him, only him.

"You'll be okay," he attempted to reassure me.

"How do you know?" I could not be convinced. Even if I were "okay," would I ever really be "okay" again? Knowing that I had my health and that he did not – would that be "okay?" No. This was not fair.

"So I'll go next Monday." But, in my heart, I wanted the test right then. I could hardly wait out the week for next Monday's test. And then I could not possibly be patient another two weeks for the results.

But I had to wait. The scenarios replayed in my head and terrified me.

"We'll talk in the morning." Gil marched upstairs to bed, visibly drained.

I shouted optimistically to his back as he ascended the stairs. "Everything will look different in the morning, Gil."

But there are some things a new morning cannot change.

I was up early, as usual, getting ready for work while Gil was still in bed. Drinking coffee, I watched the birds outside at our feeder and noticed the buds showing color and swelling on the crabapple tree and lilac bush. The landscape – grasses, trees, and gardens – was rebounding from winter's cruelty. Would we also rebound?

Gil pattered down the stairs. It was unusual to see him so early in the morning. He was never awake before I left for work.

"Need a warmup for that coffee?" he asked.

"No, I'm fine." I still had no words I could say to him, or so I thought.

"I'll be right in to join you."

I was not used to being with Gil so early in the morning. This quiet time of day had evolved over the past four years into my private time. Was Gil intruding on my sanctuary? How could I be so possessive of time, a dwindling luxury?

"Look at the bird feeder, Gil," were the only words I could say to him. "The robins have come back to town."

He stared out the window and nodded. "I know what that means."

I immediately knew what he meant. Gil's favorite time of year, the warm weather months, was approaching. He would once again lounge on a deck chair before going into work after his lunch, perfecting his tan. Or would he? The anxious scenarios began to replay in my mind: *Might this summer be spent in and out of hospitals? Will he be taking photosensitive medications prohibiting sun exposure?*

Will he even see this summer?

"Gil, let's talk about what we need to do." What did we need to do? Anything, yet? I had no answers. I did not even know my health status. What if I was also sick? *Maybe he will outlive me?* "You know, I may not even be around to take care of you."

"No conversation today," Gil cut short the movie in my mind. I had lived long enough with this man to know when it was time to let something go.

My words of neutrality and normalcy returned. "Let's just enjoy the robins this morning, Gil."

Andrew's Test

February 1991

The following Monday night was my turn to go to the health center, alone. For the first time, the preliminary consulting session seemed more intensive than any of the many times I had been through it before. Or was I merely paying more attention?

"Have you been engaging in any sexual activities that you think might have put you at risk for HIV infection?" asked the peer counselor, Alice.

"Yes."

"Do you use protection during sex?"

"No."

"Are you in a relationship?"

"Yes."

"How long have you been a couple?" She attempted to make my one word replies into sentences.

"Four years." It must have been working; I answered with two words.

"Monogamous?"

"Yes." Back to the one-word replies. *Monogamous as far as I know.* I believed it to be so. But I would never ask Gil... afraid of his answer. I needed to believe it to be so.

Her last question triggered the scenarios as I sat opposite her, silently debating whether I should continue going through with the test or get up and leave. Despite my yearly routine testing and somewhat broad knowledge of the virus, Gil and I had never used a condom during our four years together. *Why not?* That simple question confirmed the results of the anticipated test. I, too, must be HIV-positive. Why bother to wait the two-week period for the lab's confirmation? Why did it still take a two-week timeframe from blood sampling to test results? One would think the test would have been perfected and streamlined in the years it had been in existence.

"Are you particularly concerned about your HIV status at this time?"

"Of course. My partner was confirmed HIV-positive last week." My voice crackled as I said it aloud for first time, and to a stranger.

"Did your partner come here for his test?" Alice asked.

"Yes."

"Did he come back for a second confirmation test?"

"No. He wasn't given that option. The test came back positive."

"I must confess. Your partner was the first person I had to inform was HIV-positive since working here. I guess I was so shaken by the reality of the result that I neglected to tell him to come in for a second confirmation test."

I processed her disclosure. Was AIDS so isolated in New Hampshire in 1991 that this was her first positive confirmation? I would probably be the second person with whom she would have to share such news within a two-week period. Alice would be a pro at it in no time. I was angry. Not at Alice. Not at Gil. At the virus.

"I'll let him know he has that option." At that point I realized I also had a choice. Now would be the perfect time for me to stand, tell Alice I had changed my mind, and apologize for taking up her valuable time. A nurse had drawn no blood, and a costly test had not yet been performed by some unidentified laboratory – I could walk away now. No harm done to anyone. Except me.

But because I was here and had taken the time to sit through her preliminary counseling, I might as well have the blood drawn. After all, being anonymous, I was under no obligation to return for the results. Or was I bound to myself and to Gil to follow through with it?

"You may come back in two weeks for the results. I'll see you then."

Two weeks of limbo.

Two weeks of being able to think of nothing but the pronouncement of the upcoming positive test results.

Two weeks of reliving my past, asking myself repeatedly: *Why didn't we?* Questioning daily whether our relationship had been monogamous; and, if so, how many years before I met Gil had he been infected with HIV? Where did Gil pick it up?

Did I even need answers to these questions?

Two weeks of thinking about how I would care for Gil, with me also being HIV-positive. Could he care for me, if necessary? Who would become sick first? Who would die first? Who had the answers?

Two weeks of tortured thoughts. Meditations kept to myself. Selfish prayers for a negative test result, however unlikely.

The two weeks inched by. Alice, no longer a stranger, once again sat opposite me for the consultation. This visit, I had given her my first name. She now had information too important to treat me as an anonymous number.

"Andrew, I have great news." Alice's tone of voice had not been so emotionally charged during our first meeting, two weeks earlier.

"I'm HIV-negative?" I asked incredulously.

"Yes." Her one-word response confounded my disbelief.

How could that be? HIV was a virus running wild in the gay community. Add to that fact, during our four years of intimacy, a condom had never come between Gil and me. How could I have lived so intimately with this killing virus in my home and not be infected? Only affected?

"How do you plan to take care of yourself? To take care of your partner?" Alice saw my mind wandering.

"My partner's name is Gil. He's HIV-positive. And I don't know the answers."

"Did Gil come back for a second confirmation test?"

"No."

"He can return for a free second test."

"I'll let him know, Alice." But I was sure he would not return.

Enough anonymity. Enough of having answers. Enough of HIV/AIDS invading my life, our lives. Enough.

Nervously, I expected Gil's nightly, 7:30 check-in phone call and realized our roles had been reversed in just two short weeks. I now had to tell him my HIV status over the telephone.

The ringing brought me back to the moment, back from those recurring scenarios.

"So?" without a greeting and with only one word, Gil dove into the heart of our conversation.

"Negative." No delayed buildup on my part. To the point. Possibly apologetic.

"That's so great." His voice relayed enthusiasm, sincerity, and love.

Great? Great for whom? Great for me? So that I can have a long, lonely, healthy life of always feeling guilty for not also being infected? Great for you? So that I can always be there for you through the end?

"I guess you could call it great," I replied.

Would I be there for him through the end? I knew nothing about taking care of someone who was dying. I was thirty-six years old. I should not have to be dealing with this so early in my life, only four years into our relationship. Gil also was thirty-six, and he should not have to face dying so early in his life, so early into our relationship. Caregiving should be destined for the elderly. Death should be the natural departure from this life when we are in our eighties or nineties, not in our thirties. I was angry.

"Gil, we'll talk more when you get home." I needed to get off the phone. I felt guilty about my growing doubts.

"Okay. But we need to think about what comes next."

———————

Within the week, I suggested we visit the local non-profit AIDS agency. My immediate concern was to get Gil's medical support system in place before we actually would need one. They provided the name of the one and only infectious disease doctor practicing in our area and a package of information, contacts, and support groups for those whose lives were infected and affected by HIV/AIDS. Our lives. Our hidden-from-the-world lives.

As I waited for Gil in the doctor's reception room, I looked over the package of AIDS information. One brochure specifically caught my attention: "BECOME A BUDDY." Maybe if I went through a training process, I could become better prepared to be Gil's personal "buddy"–Gil's caregiver. Maybe I could practice being a buddy for someone else until Gil needed me in this role. At that time, I would be an experienced buddy, a caregiver who knew exactly what to do. I felt so unprepared for this role.

Gil emerged from the doctor's examining room with a serious look on his face.

"My T-cell count is under 200. That means I have AIDS. Guess I slept through HIV."

Gil was closer to death than either of us had imagined.

When we returned home I called the AIDS agency. Yes, they would mail me the buddy program application, which arrived soon after. Ten pages of application forms to be completed, a request for three written letters of reference, tuberculosis test result confirmation, and driver's insurance verification. The application paperwork seemed overwhelming. I merely wanted to learn how to take care of Gil. With all the questions to answer and the requested references and tests, I felt as though I were singly reapplying for a mortgage all over again. It should not be so difficult to become a buddy, a caregiver.

I focused on the scheduled training dates — two weekend retreats in October. The two weekends Gil and I planned to be on vacation in Florida. I could not take the training sessions, even if I overcame the insurmountable amount of preliminary paperwork. Resigned, I pushed it all aside and thought of our upcoming trip to Disney World. *What if this was to be our last vacation together?*

Six months later we were in Disney World. For those six months we denied death. Our only reminders were the AIDS medications that now accompanied Gil everywhere, all the time.

September 1993

Two years later, we were once again in Disney World. Morphine had replaced AZT and ddC as the drug of choice. Gil no longer wanted the trial medications. Morphine now masked the pain of neuropathy, an irreversible side effect of the AZT/ddC drug combination. Upon returning home from possibly his last trip to Florida, Gil headed upstairs, visibly tired, and I grabbed the most recent newspaper to find out what had been happening in town during our absence. Tucked away in the community events section was a small paragraph soliciting volunteers for Strafford Hospice Care. Wasn't hospice an option we wanted to eventually investigate? I immediately called the listed number, ready to sign on.

After a few minutes of in-depth conversation with Arlene, the volunteer coordinator, she announced, "I'm sorry, Andrew. This particular program is geared for people who have already experienced a loss, not for those actively going through the process."

I could not believe what I was hearing. I was not yet "going through the process," or so I thought. Gil was not actively dying. He was merely tired and on pain medication. Hospice would not help me prepare for Gil's death?

She attempted to justify her reasons for not allowing me to become a volunteer.

"Some of the information during training may be too overwhelming for what's going on in your life."

"But Arlene, you don't understand. Gil is not yet dying. He goes to work every day. We lead normal lives. And I need to be prepared for what is coming. We're not 'going through' anything at this time. Why can't I learn about hospice, about caregiving, about what is going to happen to us?" I rapidly fired my thoughts at her.

"I'm sorry." She tried to silence me with her rules. "We have our philosophies, policies, and procedures."

"If that's the way it is..." I was ready to slam down the receiver. Enough.

"Andrew, don't hesitate to call us if you need any of our services at any time."

As if I would call again. Didn't she understand I was looking for one of their services right now?

"We want to be here for you." Her voice droned on.

Well you're not. Can't you see that?

"Thanks for your time, Arlene. I understand your position." I did NOT understand her position. I had reached for help and had not received what I needed. I felt alone. Was this the introduction to what I would face throughout this entire caregiving ordeal? Isolation? Rejection? Non-support? Inadequate caregiving knowledge?

As I spent the next hour trying to figure out what I could do to prepare myself for this frightening caregiving role, the phone rang.

"Andrew?"

I recognized the voice.

"It's Arlene from Hospice."

"Hello again." *What more could you possibly have to say to me?*

"I've discussed your specific situation with our team, and we've reconsidered your circumstances and our position."

"And?" Could there have been a change since our conversation just one hour ago?

"Our nine-week volunteer training course starts this Saturday. Will you join us?"

"I'll be there."

Hope squashed anger, anxiety, and hysteria. Now I had a sense of direction. I would become a trained hospice volunteer – Gil's personal "hospice buddy."

See Appendix A: End-of-Life Coaching Exercise...
TWO QUESTIONS, page 245.

"MY WORLD IS EMPTY WITHOUT YOU"

Hospice Volunteer Training
Session One:
Personal Loss Inventories

The 1993 Fall Volunteer Training Course will start on Saturday, September 18th with an all-day session to be held at a local hospital. The eight remaining sessions will be held on the next eight Monday evenings from 5:30 p.m. to 8:00 p.m.

The training sessions are designed to prepare volunteers in a variety of areas, including listening and communications skills, medical management, grief and bereavement, spiritual needs, funeral customs, and community resources.

The notice for the training session performed somersaults between my fingers as I worried about my readiness for Saturday's all-day session. Was hospice the final care decision we would ultimately choose? It should of course be Gil's decision, and he knew as little about hospice as I. Was he even ready to talk about this end-of-life option? My concept of hospice's philosophy was treating the whole person and not just the disease. Hospice workers came into your home to make everyday living with disease more comfortable for the patient and provide support for the family. It was a team of health care professionals and volunteers making that happen.

"Hospice" connoted for me a feeling of warm caring, contrasting sharply with the cold invasiveness of hospital care. I needed to know for both of us if Gil would receive end-of-life services at home and if we would find the necessary medical, social, physical, and emotional supports we would need. In only nine sessions, would I receive the training to become an adequate caregiver? Would hospice extend into the murky period following Gil's death? Were we eligible for hospice care? What would it cost? I had many questions to bring to that first session.

September 1993

Early Saturday morning, I was in a room with ten strangers with whom I would be spending the entire day. Arlene, the volunteer coordinator, facilitated the training; and she was as animated in person as she had been on the telephone. I could not stop staring at her asymmetrical, mushroom-shaped hairstyle. It was so much safer to focus on her hair than to make eye contact with the strangers in the room.

We introduced ourselves, and Arlene presented us with the hospice's history, organization, and philosophy. She described the expectations for trainees and volunteers. We spent the entire day doing Personal

Death Awareness Inventories — sharing the losses in our lives that had brought us together for this hospice volunteer training. It evolved into a day of intense sharing of grief that spanned years.

I was mourning the anticipated future loss of Gil, and of our future; but in this room, I discovered that a loss need not be death and that it may affect someone for a very long time, perhaps throughout the remainder of a person's life. I heard intimate stories of losses of career due to age; of a breast to cancer; of the witnessing of the drowning of a brother during childhood; and of the losses of parents, spouses, children, friends, and pets. Every recounted tale was a past event with lifelong residual effects, comparable with my current fear of upcoming loss.

We began our final exercise of the first session, in which each of us was to write the five most important things in our life on five separate pieces of paper. I scribbled "GIL," "HEALTH," "HOME," "FAMILY," and "CAREER." We were told to tear up one of the five sheets of paper — which one would it be? If you had to lose just one of the five most cherished parts of your life, which one could you do without most comfortably? I chose to lose "CAREER." It was an agonizing exercise in loss by choice. Such things in life usually do not become a choice. How could our lives go on comfortably without incomes? *Should I have torn one of the other four options?*

"Now tear another," said Arlene.

"FAMILY."

"And another."

"HOME."

"One more."

"HEALTH."

A brief video of a hospice patient and family followed the exercise. It portrayed the ideal situation in which the volunteer seemed to be as close as family, and the patient's death was an anticipated natural and peaceful event. *But how could this be?*

Finally, fifteen minutes of guided imagery and processing prepared us to leave the session and reenter the world. I left the room with a greater understanding of the many losses that affect people, and I was not alone.

Once home, I reviewed the assigned homework, due the next session: "Prepare a Lifeline Graph."

I retrieved the syllabus of the eight upcoming two-and-one-half-hour evening sessions to see what was yet to come. The topic titles were:

- *September 20: Introduction to Death and Dying; Patient, Family, and Children*

- *September 27: Medical Management; AIDS*

- *October 4: Communications and Listening Skills I*

- *October 11: Legal Issues; Spiritual Panel*

- *October 18: Listening Skills and Grief; Funerals*

- *October 25: Communications and Listening Skills II; Grief and Loss*

- *November 1: Comfort Measures; Managing Personal Stress; and Termination*

- *November 8: Policies and Procedures; Volunteer Panel; Graduation*

Maybe I should start the homework assignment while the topics were fresh in my mind. With a ruler, I drew a straight line on a blank sheet of bright, white paper. At the line origin on the left, I entered "March 12, 1954, I am born." At the end on the right, I projected "March 12, 1994, 40 Years of Age – My World is Shattered." Tears blurred the image of the line. I began to think of lifecycle events that had happened during my forty years, and of the ones that now would never transpire.

Determined to carry the assignment to the finish, I filled in "October 28, 1987, 33 Years of Age – I met Gil Victor Ornelas" and "February 15, 1991, 37 Years of Age – Gil's Diagnosis." Had there been anything else in my life of so much importance to chronicle? Shouldn't the line have extended further than March 12, 1994? Surely my life is not going to come to an end on that date. My thoughts were broken by the sound of Gil returning home from a day of shopping the outlet stores, passing the time while I was at the all-day training session.

"So how was the class?" Gil immediately asked.

"In two words, very intense."

"Dinner started?"

"No. I got wrapped up in some of the stuff from the day." I wanted to talk about the day's training session with him, not about whether dinner had been started.

"So let me show you the turtlenecks that were on sale at Eddie Bauer."

I stared at him in disbelief.

"Look at these great colors."

Gil, I want to tell you what I experienced today.

Shoving the oversized plastic bag in my direction, he announced,

"Here, this has the ones in your size."

Don't you get it, Gil? We need to share this. Together. I can't do it alone.

"Hope the colors aren't too *cha-cha* for you."

I realize you don't want to know any more of my all-day hospice volunteer training after hearing the two words "very intense." But that will change with time. It has to.

"I'll start dinner while you try on those shirts." He rummaged through the refrigerator for salad ingredients.

I went upstairs to try on a half dozen turtlenecks in gaudy, "cha-cha" colors that I never would have chosen for myself.

See Appendix B: End-of-Life Coaching Exercise...
PERSONAL LOSS INVENTORY, page 246.

See Appendix C: End-of-Life Coaching Exercise...
LIFELINE GRAPH, page 247.

March 30, 1996

I sat on the edge of the adjustable bed thinking of appropriate activities. We never discussed what was to happen during this time, these four hours he requested I spend alone with him once he died. Our house seemed so empty and peaceful now.

"Gil, I want to lie next to you and hold you in my arms one last time." *But I need to do more, our last entire morning together.* "I'll save that for just before it's time for you to leave." I felt so physically drained as I talked to him.

"There's nothing more I can say that you haven't already heard." I had shared with him the emotional floods as I experienced them this past month. I also felt so mentally drained.

"I've told you, Gil, how much I love you and how brave you are. I've assured you that I'll be all right, and that you have my permission to go, that it is time to go." I have said "I forgive you," "please forgive me," and "thank you." He did not need to hear any more of this from me.

I took care of Gil these last four years. I did not remember what else there might be for me to do this morning, now that I no longer had that function. I left his bedside long enough to light the heather-scented votive candle I had placed on the table next to his bed. Gil loved scented candles. I looked away from him for a moment, up toward the right angles of the room where walls meet ceiling. These corners were slightly blackened from eight years of his frequent candle burning in this living room. *I need to light this candle just one last time before he leaves.*

"Gil, do you remember that journal I gave you for your birthday two summers ago?" I gently stroked his limp, fine brown hair, once so full, curly, and black.

"You had so much time alone at home back then. I thought you might have the urge to record some of the feelings you wrestled with, regarding your illness."

He never complained to me or discussed his pain, so I thought he might be comfortable writing in a journal. Was he feeling anger? Was he denying the illness? Did he merely accept his fate and graciously make the most of each day that came along?

My fingers moved from his hair, reluctantly touching the frozen coolness of his countenance. "Gil, if you would not talk to me of your thoughts, did you record them?"

I saw him writing in that journal during a Fourth-of-July weekend, one month after receiving the cloth-bound book, and I knew the bedroom chest drawer where he always kept it. "I'm going to get your journal, and read it aloud to you now." *I need to do this with him before he leaves.*

Hoping to find many pages of expressed feelings, I was disappointed to discover only a dozen pages of his writings, spanning his thirty-ninth birthday through the ensuing three end-of-summer months. I liked looking at his open, rounded handwriting, tracing some of the letters with my finger. What I found gives me so much insight into what he did not allow himself to speak. I read of how tired he was during that time, and of how much he loves me. He wrote of how bothered he was by his family's reaction to his illness and their increasing distancing from him. He loved cooking, and the journal pages revealed his documenting and critiquing of meals shared with friends during those three months. He expressed things in those few pages that he never spoke of with me. I felt insight, but I also felt cheated because we were not able to talk of these things together. *I need to have this discussion with him now before he leaves.*

Did I hear Gil speaking? His "words" released me from thoughts of journal writings and gave me direction.

"Andrew, you now need to take care of yourself." Where was that familiar voice coming from?

"Go into the kitchen and fix yourself some breakfast." Gil seemed to warn me that three of our four allotted morning hours had passed, and the men from the funeral home would be there shortly to take him away from me.

I mechanically wandered to the kitchen and prepared scrambled eggs, toast with peanut butter and cinnamon-apple jelly, and a slice of seedless watermelon. I juiced a concoction of sliced apples, carrots, and ginger. This was Gil's favorite morning meal, one I had prepared numerous times these past four years, half of our too-brief history together. Through the kitchen window, I saw a robin perching on the now bare but soon-to-be-budding lilac bush. He cocked his head, warbled a brief melody, and returned my penetrating look through the windowpane. The first robin of spring gave me immediate awareness of time and of life continuing outside our quiet home. I must finish my breakfast and return to Gil's bedside. Our morning together had almost come to an end. I felt an excruciating need to spend as much time as I could with him before he left.

"Gil, I want to preserve this morning in some permanent way. Would you mind if I got your camera and took a picture of you?" He looked so peaceful lying in the bed, with the stuffed black bear snuggled within the frozen crook of his arm. "Would you mind if I cut a lock of your hair?"

I located the camera that was always by his side, so he could capture the moments of his final years. The photos I took that morning of Gil, who looked to me so beautiful and peaceful, would later startlingly reveal the true ravages of his disease, deteriorations of his body and mind I lovingly overlooked. However, that day I did not see the reality of his decline, because the still-emanating inner beauty of this man who died with so much grace and gentleness masked it.

Later, the developed photos would finally make me see a wasted physiognomy, his once handsome face overrun with the bumps of molluscum and blotched by the dark stains of Karposi Sarcoma. Also, the lock of baby-fine brown hair, which I cut with his sewing scissors and tied with a strand of rainbow-striped ribbon, would also later make me see the side effects of the numerous medications he took. *I need to do these intimate things while I still have the chance, before he leaves.*

"I'll honor all your requests, Gil." I would carry out his wishes for cremation, no funeral service, but rather a Celebration of Life three months later, on his birthday. He asked that I spend this half a day alone with him before being taken away. Until this morning, I never fully understood this request of four hours alone with him. I remember when he told me of his fear of being taken away and cremated while still alive, that these four hours alone with me would verify he was indeed no longer breathing. Along with taking care of Gil's anxieties, this morning with him allowed me time for reflection and for doing spontaneous things – lighting the candle, reading his journal, preparing his breakfast, taking his picture, and cutting a lock of his hair. "Thank you, Gil, for giving me this morning with you."

Fifteen minutes of our time alone remained. I climbed onto the hospital bed in our living room one last time and tightly held his unyielding body. *This embrace will need to last my lifetime.* The doorbell interrupted our final closeness. I admitted the two men from the mortuary.

"I don't want him to leave this house in a zippered plastic bag. Please, take him out with this quilt to keep him warm. And don't cover his face. I want him to feel the sun one more time." The men respected my blurted wishes.

I stood at the kitchen window once again. This time I watched as they wheeled Gil into the dark-colored funeral coach. The time had come for him to leave. I knew the March sun felt good on his face one last time. The coach drove away, and the robin once again landed on the lilac.

Now the house was truly empty.

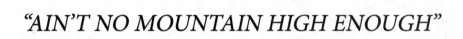

"AIN'T NO MOUNTAIN HIGH ENOUGH"

Hospice Volunteer Training
Session Two:
Coping

Eight Monday Nights of Fall 1993

I spent two and one-half hours in a hospital conference room for eight consecutive Monday nights, completing the circle of chairs on which perched a nurse, a therapist, a lawyer, and a real estate agent. We were a group from all walks of life, ranging in age from thirty to sixty. Eye contact was no longer an issue for me; we had shared too much about ourselves last Saturday, resulting in a simultaneous group bonding by day's end.

While I attended these evening hospice trainings, Gil was at work, manning the telephone as a second-shift customer service representative. He politely received calls from irritable customers whose power had been turned off, usually due to nonpayment for electric services. Upon his late evening returns, he greeted me with the same weekly question, "So how was training?"

I found that as the eight weeks progressed, so did Gil's interest and mutual participation in the many diverse topics – uncharted lands of loss and death, destinations most explorers would voluntarily circumvent. Yet this was to be our voyage. Together.

After we danced around Gil's diagnosis for eighteen months, these hospice training sessions were beginning to open the necessary communications between us, regarding some of the important issues we were yet to encounter.

September 20, 1993

The second session discussion began with Elisabeth Kübler-Ross' five stages of coping with grief: Denial. Anger. Bargaining. Depression. Acceptance.

In what stage was Gil? Could I possibly be in one of these stages? If so, which one?

Our group conversation progressed to children and how they are often left out of the dying process, in an attempt to shield them from the truth and potential emotional upset. Because there were no children involved in our scenario, my mind wandered back to those five stages.

In what stage is Gil? Denial? He is two and one-half years into his HIV diagnosis; and he is outwardly healthy.

In what stage am I? Acceptance? Isn't that why I am enrolled in hospice training?

Or Anger? Yes, I could acknowledge anger as an emotion deeply suppressed within me.

And can more than one stage be experienced simultaneously? Are these stages not ordered to fall in some logically predetermined chronology?

Hearing the words "family dynamics" brought me back into the group's discussion.

"The family system as an entity is greater than the sum of its parts," Arlene suggested to the group.

So who are the parts that make up the whole in our story?

My family of origin consisted of only my parents and me. They lived one hour north in Portland, Maine, and they had "accepted" my alternate lifestyle fourteen years prior with, "We may not approve of it, but as long as you are happy...."

Gil's family was comprised of his mother and an older half-brother. They lived an equal distance away west in New Hampshire. Gil's out-lifestyle at an earlier age, with him leaving home before finishing high school and living in distant cities such as San Francisco or Miami, miles away from his family in Kansas City, had made his homosexuality more easily "accepted" by his mother. She did not have to confront it.

Gil also had a half-sister on the West Coast, separated by thousands of miles. Gil had spoken with her only once in the few years we had been together. I knew nothing about her, other than his description of her vagrant lifestyle.

"The family system is a composite of both individual family members and their multiple interactions with one another," Arlene's voice briefly drew me back, only to be lost once again by the word "interactions."

Interactions? The verbal altercations I have witnessed during the past three years were not healthy family "interactions" as exhibited by Gil's side of the family.

"Closed family systems are characterized by prohibitions on communicating or commenting about family rules and beliefs," Arlene's squawky voice, directing the group's discussion, drew me back once again.

"Closed family systems" is a mild term for what I have observed in Gil's family concerning HIV/AIDS. "Denial, Denial, Denial" was the mantra I assumed they used to begin and end each of their days since learning of Gil's diagnosis.

And will Gil's family be there for him right through the end? I had doubts. I could easily interchange the nouns "Gil's mother" with "a child" as we continued our debate on children and death.

I was not prepared to shield, or offer the opportunity to spare, his family from emotional trauma. My anger was reemerging. Gil's mother seemed to be distancing herself well enough on her own, and I desperately needed her to acknowledge the situation, to support us, and to help me prepare for Gil's death – her own son's death. If I was not to be exempt, why should she? She had brought Gil into this world; it would be only natural that she should also take some responsibility in the preparation for his leaving our lives. *I don't think I can do this alone.*

"Next week's homework assignment is to draw a picture of your family." Our evening was coming to a close with Arlene's assignment of homework.

One last time, that evening's announcement brought me back to the group, away from disturbing thoughts of Gil's mother.

On the blank sheet of paper before me, I hastily completed the assignment on the spot, rather than wrestle with it at home.

I began my artwork, which quickly took on a life of its own. A large heart, two circles of equal size, and one small square. The heart enveloped the names "Gil and Andrew." The two circles overlapped the heart independently. One circle was designated "My Parents;" the other, "Our Friends." In a far away corner on the page was the small isolated square. Within its walls were confined the words "Gil's Family." I put the completed assignment in my notebook and headed home with many conflicting thoughts of family and death surging to the surface of my awareness. I also recognized anger as a primary player in this game of Life, with rules so different from the familiar board game of the same name I had played during my sheltered childhood.

"So how was training?" Gil asked two hours later, slamming the front door against a blast of the chilled October air.

Into the night, Gil and I discussed Kübler-Ross' five stages of grief. But I could not bring myself to mention my disturbing thoughts of his family.

See Appendix D: End-of-Life Coaching Exercise...
YOUR FAMILY, page 247.

Two Barometers

I thought Sam could be the barometer to gauge the upcoming calms and storms of Gil's disease, but I could not accurately predict the weather patterns of terminal illness. I learned it is futile to compare one person's dying with another's.

Our neighbor, Janet, had a son, Sam, in his mid-forties. Janet, Gil, and I did not yet know that Sam had a secret. Sam was HIV-positive, and he had been for years. "Dying" was a word not yet in Sam's vocabulary. In the recesses of his mind, Sam wanted to spare his mother the pain and the potential embarrassment associated with an AIDS death. Sam was in denial; AIDS was his secret, and financial circumstances forced Sam home to live with his mother.

After we knew him for a year, Sam finally revealed his secret to Gil and me.

"Guys, I need to tell you that I'm HIV-positive." Sam blurted out this information in the middle of a conversation with us. "But don't tell anyone."

"Does your mother know?" Gil asked, knowing the answer.

"No." He shot back a look of *Don't you even think of telling her.*

"Are you planning to tell her?"

"No." Sam was adamant in his response. "Not until I need to."

"I told my mother when I found out," Gil offered, sounding somewhat boastful. "She seemed to handle it okay." Gil attempted reasoning. "Even though we don't talk about it, always around it."

"My mother's different. She's already been through too much family stuff." Sam had an excuse. "I can't burden her with this."

"But my mother lost a son in Vietnam, and she has outlived a few of her husbands over the years." Gil again attempted to persuade Sam to tell his mother. "And she's coping."

"I just can't do it to my mother." Sam was not going to reconsider.

"Sam, you're living with your mother." I finally joined in on their conversation, still in shock of having something revealed to me that I had suspected for the past year "How can you hide it from her?"

"I've known for years." It was clear Sam was not going to tell his mother.

"Okay, Sam. Whatever works for you. Just remember, you can talk to us about it anytime."

That night, as I washed our dinner dishes, I thought about Sam and Gil as weather barometers. Maybe I could track and plot Gil's eventual decline against Sam's. It might be less painful for me to watch death slightly removed – through Sam. There were similarities between Sam and Gil. Both were working full time, both driving cars, both eating whatever they chose, and both taking myriad medications in ever-changing quantities and varieties. Sam, at this time, seemed as outwardly healthy as Gil; yet they both harbored the same disease. Shortly, all these factors would change.

There were differences. Gil's medical care was local, and he was covered under his employer's medical plan; Sam's care was a free health clinic an hour away in Boston where he would receive trial drugs or, possibly and unknowingly, a placebo. Most importantly, Gil's disease was now public knowledge; Sam's diagnosis was his secret.

That evening, both men registered "calm" on the barometer's gauge.

For months following Sam's revelation, both men lived simple, seemingly healthy lives. After three months passed, Gil made the decision to go on disability leave from his job. He could no longer physically tolerate the hour commute each way or deal with the stress of high-volume customer complaints on the phone. To me, Gil looked much the same, only weary. In reality, he had lost close to twenty five pounds and had a newly acquired hovering anxiousness. Fatigue, both physical and mental, were his major concerns.

When Gil made his disability-leave decision, he felt he had only months to live. Sam was still energetic, while Gil was visibly tired. I watched Sam make repeated trips to Boston to be fitted for a wig to vainly cover his naturally balding head, and I watched Gil lose a full head of curly hair as a result of his medications.

Gil acknowledged AIDS and death with the dignity of quiet acceptance, whereas Sam remained in a secret world of raging denial. Their weather of disease changed sporadically. Physically, Gil registered "stormy," but "calm" mentally. Sam seemed just the opposite.

The foliage began to color, and both barometers' needles reflected the changes. Sam and Gil hibernated indoors for warmth and spent their communal time sharing stories of the latest medications' side effects, foods they could no longer tolerate, and the length of the day's nap. That summer, Sam informed his mother he was HIV-positive, never calling it AIDS. Mother and son now shared Sam's secret, and both were in denial. In contrast, Gil and his mother had known of Gil's diagnosis for three years. During this time, Gil was in acceptance, while Gil's mother resembled Sam and Janet in their denial. I had fully accepted Gil's disease since the diagnosis, and I had started to mourn both Sam and Gil.

That winter both barometers read "stormy." Sam refused to give up driving; to keep him and others on the road safe, his mother resorted to hiding his car keys. I watched Sam's bald head swell from a lymphoma in the brain, the area of his body where the AIDS virus destructively manifested itself. His no-longer-fitting wig was tossed on his bedside bureau. Sam's belly painfully rounded from the medications' side effects, his gait faltered, his mind wandered, and his stare became vacant.

I refused to acknowledge these same traits in Gil as we purchased his jeans in steadily increasing waist sizes, before switching over to elasticized sweatpants. I patiently listened as he started stories that somehow always lost their endings.

As the 1994 winter holiday season approached, Gil believed it would be his last. We decided that Christmas would be a day alone in our home with no intrusions from friends or family. This was a selfish indulgence we deemed necessary because, just doors away, Sam's rapidly declining health served as a daily reminder of Gil's own condition. Our holiday home was peaceful as we dined together and exchanged gifts. In contrast, Sam's holiday household was in turmoil. Sam's care was no longer manageable by his mother and the recently hired visiting nurses. Sam's brother from New Jersey announced Christmas Day that Sam could no longer stay at home with their mother – his care was becoming too demanding. He made this known amidst their not-so-festive day of Sam's confusion, repeated bathing, and instability.

Sam's brother interrupted our quiet holiday celebration to ask if he could bring Sam to visit while he, his mother, and other brother gathered for an emergency meeting. They needed to determine what direction to follow with Sam's rapidly declining condition. I had witnessed Sam's recent deterioration and knew I could not have Gil watching and breathing death so closely on Christmas Day. I answered Sam's brother with a firm "No," adding that I strongly believed any family decisions concerning Sam should be made with Sam present.

I knew I could never make such a final decision without Gil being present, whether or not he was able to contribute to the decision making. For the second time that Christmas Day, I felt selfish. Yet I remained firm. I needed to protect Gil and to allow him the perfect day, as this Christmas could be his last. Sam's mother had planned their holiday around Sam being home for one last family gathering, regardless of Sam's condition, and it turned out to be a final holiday with few pleasant memories for any of them.

Sam's family had their meeting while Sam slept in his bedroom upstairs. Their conclusion: he would be taken to a hospital for observation. A few days at the hospital determined that nothing more could be done for Sam, and he was transferred to the hospice wing of a nearby rehabilitation center.

During those days following Christmas, Gil and I visited Sam in the hospital and then one last time at the rehab center on the night before we left for a month-long winter sojourn to South Carolina. If only I could have read Gil's mind as he sat holding Sam's hand, gently stroking his arm. Gil spoke softly to Sam of their escapades over the past two years, recalling stories I had not been privy to until that bedside evening. Many of them revolved around a vacation to Key West both men had taken only months before. Gil reminisced about the horrendous day of plane travel they both barely tolerated and how tired they were once they arrived. They spent their week sitting poolside, too tired to venture downtown for shopping and their stomachs too upset by medications to dine out.

Hearing these misadventures recounted made me feel left out of this small episode in Gil's life and made me realize that I would, once again, be abandoned by both these men when they took their final journeys, this time traveling separately.

Sam's only recognition of our presence in the room was in his eyes, slowly moving back and forth from Gil's face to mine. Sam did not speak in response to Gil's soothing voice. I sat at the foot of Sam's bed and watched Gil assume the role of caregiver, comforting our friend as they both died of AIDS according to their own allotted timetables. My future flashed before me as I heard Gil whisper, "It's okay to let go, Sam."

Had Sam been Gil's barometer or his mirror? I looked at the two men, side by side, one last time. That night, the three of us sat in the eye of the storm of AIDS. Gil's barometer misleadingly read "calm."

Sam's no longer registered any information. Sam died two days later. Gil lived to celebrate one more Christmas.

"STOP! IN THE NAME OF LOVE"

Hospice Volunteer Training
Session Three:
Cancer and AIDS

September 27, 1993

Two guest speakers were scheduled for the evening's hospice training: an oncology nurse and a person living with AIDS.

The nurse, Charlotte, began the presentation. She recounted her cancer nursing stories, each case spanning from diagnosis to death, touching on the patient's initial reaction to the news and how the cancer patient usually found eventual acceptance and peace before death. Charlotte also spoke of some families' reactions to the diagnosis and the ensuing, customarily invasive treatment – case histories ranging from total family support to spousal abandonment.

Abandonment? I could never leave Gil over this. Be honest, Andrew, had the thought never entered your head? Of course, maybe once. Or twice.

But Gil and I had made a commitment to each other. So there was no honorable easy way out. Gil's exit was through death, and I prayed it would come peacefully. That, in itself, was not a guaranteed easy way out. I expected to be there right to the end, as I would have expected Gil to be there for me had our fates been reversed.

The recently recognized Anger within me began to churn as I heard Charlotte detail the story of a husband who left his wife after her mastectomy, feeling she was no longer a whole woman.

No, I vowed to myself, *regardless of how difficult this will be for Gil and for me, I am not walking out on Gil. Never. Ever.*

She ended her talk with witnessed events. Firsthand stories sharing the moments of death of some of her patients. Charlotte, a nurse whose career centered on cancer, described in detail the final processes of the body's shutdown in either of two planes: the physical and the emotional/spiritual/mental.

Charlotte described the physical symptoms: coolness of the skin; increased sleeping or changes in consciousness; restlessness or anxiety; fluid and food decrease; urine and bowel changes; physical pain; disorientation; incontinence; changes in breathing; and rare incidents of seizures, choking, or bleeding.

Which of these will I experience with Gil? I am not medically trained to deal with any such symptoms. Can I do this?

She also elaborated on the emotional/spiritual/mental symptoms: near-death awareness experiences; anxiety or restlessness; decreased socialization; unusual communication; giving permission; and saying goodbye.

Which of these would I experience in the process? Probably all. And yet I felt more comfortable with this plane of symptoms. Maybe I

COULD do this.

My eyes sought support from others in the room. Unlike me, this group had intimately known cancer throughout their lives. On the other hand, I did not believe anyone in this group experienced AIDS as omnipresently in their lives as I did. To me, cancer meant taking a foreign trip; AIDS meant staying at home.

After a short break, the session continued with a person living with AIDS, accompanied by a trained hospice "volunteer buddy." A man and a woman entered our intimate conference space. To our predominantly heterosexual group, the man must have been the quintessential "gay man with AIDS." He was of frail structure, articulate speech with the hint of a lisp, impeccable dress, and multiple gold earrings puncturing one earlobe and continuing up the ear's rim of cartilage. The woman appeared to be the privileged "all-American housewife" with ample time in her life to do charitable volunteer work, so she presumably chose to become a "buddy" for this man dying of AIDS.

The woman spoke first.

"Good evening. My name is Connie and I'm HIV-positive."

I felt the thick, hot undercurrents of expelled air as I watched the disbelief on the faces of my peer volunteer trainees. AIDS, unlike cancer, was not their world, except for the information they got from the media. A woman with AIDS had broken our preconceived stereotype, particularly as an HIV-positive woman in 1993 rural New Hampshire.

Without missing a beat, and in defiance of the visible disbelief she encountered, Connie continued her introduction. "And this is my 'buddy,' David. He is a wonderfully supportive gay man who is HIV-negative. I find David to be the perfect person to spend my time with. He distracts me from the daily reality of AIDS. He knows this plague firsthand. Many of his friends are HIV-positive or have died of AIDS, and he can tap into a support community of those who are dealing or have dealt with the same issues that confront me daily: medical care, financing expensive drug treatments, discrimination, isolation, fear." Unlike the more readily accepted world of cancer, what Connie spoke of was my quiet world, and Gil's world.

The evening came to a close with a wrap-up of the presented material. Not a word was spoken about cancer; AIDS dominated our conversations. AIDS did not discriminate among those it affected. A person living with AIDS required special precautions, and we spoke of those safeguards that should be observed when working with a person with AIDS. The group also discussed the fear of contagion and the homophobia one might encounter when working with someone with AIDS.

The distribution of the homework assignment ended the session. This week's project seemed more involved than that of last week; I would need to complete this one at home.

After class, sitting at the dining room table, I looked over the task.

Homework Assignment:

1. *Your philosophy of Death. For ten uninterrupted minutes, in a diary or log, record your feelings, thoughts, beliefs, and attitudes about death while reflecting on the questions below. Don't monitor this process — do it as a stream of consciousness.*

2. *Questions: What is death?*

Why do people die?

What happens when they die or after they die?

How do you feel about your own death?

3. *When you finish, underline the most important ideas, feelings, or concepts and develop them into a short philosophy of death.*

With Gil due home in a couple of hours, I began to write, stream of consciousness:

Death is inevitable. Death is a major loss. Death at an early age is not fair. Death is final.

People die because the body eventually wears down — the normal scenario. People die because disease enters their world and prematurely breaks the body down — the abnormal scenario, our scenario, and the unfair scenario. And people die when they know it is their time to let go — when they have completed whatever mission they needed to achieve while alive. But people also die in unexpected tragic accidents, without completing their life mission during this lifetime. However, I believe in a potential for the accomplishment during another lifetime.

When people die, the body releases the "soul." I believe there are only so many "souls" out there, and when the "soul" is released upon death, it will eventually inhabit another new life form. This "soul" transference can go on for many generations until the "soul" finally "gets it right." When this happens, then the "soul" can transcend to the highest level of peace. That is why, when we meet someone new, we sometimes feel that we have already met this person. I believe that these moments are when "souls" from other lifetimes reconnect; "souls" that had at some time previously been in contact/conflict.

My own death? I want it to be peaceful and at home, and I want my "soul" to transcend to that higher level upon my death. I want to think that I finally "got it right" during this short lifetime with Gil.

The egg timer sounded its alarm after ten minutes. As I looked over my writing, I heard Gil coming through the door, slamming it shut so the latch pin connected with strike plate.

"So, what did you learn in training tonight?" His expected Monday night greeting.

"Honey, listen to this." I quickly started to read:

Death is an inevitable loss. In normal situations, death occurs when a person is both physically and spiritually ready to let go of life. Upon death, the "soul" has the opportunity to transcend to a higher level. Only death can provide that beautiful, peaceful passage of the "soul."

"So, what do you think, Gil?"

An awkward silence filled the room.

See Appendix E: End-of-Life Coaching Exercise...
PHILOSOPHY OF DEATH, page 248.

The Art of Kissing

October 1995

The Art of Kissing is a forty-seven-page paperback book measuring 5 by 7 inches by less than 1/8 inch thick. It is printed in black ink on paper with the weight, color, and feel of cheap newspaper. Copyrighted in 1936; reprinted in 1988; author, Hugh Morris. On the title page is Gil's handwriting:

> 10/95
> To: Andy
> All my love,
> Gil

I remember my feelings of inadequacy surrounding this eighth anniversary gift. Had I become distant without realizing it? I did not think so. Was he subtly trying to tell me this with a book about kissing? I hoped not. I scanned the table of contents. A sampling of some of the chapter titles were:

> *Different Kinds of Kisses*
> *Why People Kiss*
> *Why Kissing is Pleasant*

Kisses Are But Preludes to Love
Preparing for the Kiss
The Techniques of Kissing
Enjoy the Thrills of Kissing
Put Variety into Your Kisses
Variation Kisses Are the Spice of Love

Was Gil trying to tell me something with this book? No, it must have been merely a gag gift. Yet I was devastated. Throughout his illness, I thought we had maintained the intensity of a loving relationship. Was I slowly shutting down, as his illness became more visible? No, I refused to believe it. I knew my tongue no longer urgently searched his mouth during a kiss; our mouth contacts had become merely surface touchings. I thought this was a mutually accepted boundary. He had become so concerned with his personal hygiene, diligently conscious of preventing the spread of his virus. We both knew that his mouth harbored the mysteries of thrush; a cottony, fungal growth kept in check with the drug Diflucan.

It was not my caregiving duties that I questioned; it was my commitment as a loving partner that was under scrutiny. Was the intensity of my love for Gil diminishing? Of course not. Was his measure of this in a kiss? I hoped not. I recalled asking as I unwrapped the book, "Gil, are you trying to tell me something?" His reply was, "No, Honey. Everyone just needs a refresher once in a while."

Gil could be a diplomat. He later purred beside me in bed as I examined the kissing book. He had obviously spent some time looking through it before giving it to me; I found a subscription card from *Horticulture* magazine, folded in half, marking the chapter titled, "Enjoy the Thrills of Kissing." Was this as far as he had gotten reading through the book, or was he marking this specific chapter for me? I read the chapter aloud as if it were our evening's entertainment. Certain phrases lingered on my tongue as I heard them spoken in my voice: "As in all matters pertaining to love, don't hurry the process of kissing. That is why, when kissing, there should be as many contacts, bodily contacts, as possible. Forget time. Forget everything but the kiss in which you are in the midst of."

I closed the book and held the sleeping man beside me. I did not want Gil to ever leave me, yet I could feel him slipping away. Could such a simple thing as a kiss bring him back to me? Bring me back to him?

I pulled away the comforter and flannel sheets to reveal the naked man with whom I had spent eight years. Starting at the top of his head, I caressed his prescription-drug-altered hair. I kissed his scalp, wanting to restore vitality first to his hair and then to the rest of his body. I touched every inch of him as he slept. His arms no longer showed definition. I tenderly kissed both arms, remembering with closed eyes how strong they once were when holding me. Now those arms barely clung to me for support.

His chest had hollowed; there were but wisps of hair where once a dense, black forest flourished. Again, those medications seemed to destroy and not heal. I lingered kisses on his chest, hovering the longest time above the area over his heart, knowing that pulsing beneath the pale skin lay what kept him going, both emotionally and physically. So much love surged from that heart, and I needed to somehow keep it nurtured.

Repositioning my body on the bed so that I was now at its foot, I gently massaged Gil's feet. I studied his fungus-darkened toenails and the bluish tint of the spidery-veined, splotched skin surrounding his toes. The neuropathy, resulting from those trial combinations of medications, had robbed sensation to all his extremities. His weakened immune system had allowed the invasion of the fungal growth beneath his toenails. His feet were once beautiful, slender, and arched. They were now tired, contorted, and pained. My lips caressed those feet, wanting to restore their once-supportive energy.

I repeatedly stroked his now hairless, scrawny, lesion-stained legs. I was searching for any remaining muscle tone, attempting to erase every individual lesion with a kiss. Leaning back on one elbow, I surveyed the living remains of my lover's body from head to foot. I had been doing everything I could do to keep his mind and body healthy. But had I been doing enough for his heart? Crawling back to the head of the bed, I rested my head above his heart. My breath began to match his shallow, rhythmic breathing; we became one in synchronicity. His chest gently buoyed my head as my eyes were directed toward his genitals.

This area of his body had become his self-imposed no-man's land for the past four years, beginning the very night he was diagnosed with HIV. Gil felt the AIDS virus had created a loaded gun between his thighs, and, to protect me, he had banished sex from our lives. I thought we had successfully redirected our intimacy. But was that possible? When I reached over and cupped his shriveled testicles in my hand, my mind suddenly exploded with rediscovered physical passion. I wept for all the things this man had given up during his short lifetime, and I cried out with the realization of what I soon would lose.

Feeling the room's draft on my exposed shoulders, I pulled at the layers of flannel sheeting and down comforter, once again hiding our naked bodies from the night. I held Gil tightly in my arms, not yet ready to release him to anyone, especially to Death. Gil responded to my hug long enough to mumble, "Honey, that's nice. I love you so much."

The Art of Kissing was the last anniversary gift I received from Gil. Inspired by it, I made it my conscious effort, starting that night, to kiss Gil in many more ways than lips touching lips. I made certain I did this every day for the five remaining months, before I had to let him go.

"YOU KEEP ME HANGIN' ON"

Hospice Volunteer Training
Session Four:
Being Present

October 4, 1993

"It isn't what you say, but how you say it," were Arlene's opening words.

Listening skills headlined the evening's agenda.

"And oftentimes you need say nothing. Just being present to another person is the key."

Being present.

"Don't try to solve problems; allow the person to have his pain. Learn to be with the person. Don't react, respond."

Allow the person to have his pain. Such a difficult concept when you want to ease that pain.

I like to think I was following these guidelines. It was so hard. AIDS was with us twenty-four hours each day. It was not as though I were a typical volunteer buddy who spent two hours, twice a week with a person with AIDS. It consumed our every thought. *Don't react, respond?* How could I respond if we spoke about it only infrequently? Our at-home communication was just beginning to evolve with these weekly training sessions, but there did not seem to be enough reality discussion going on. *Don't react?* I knew she was talking locally and not globally, to the person, not the disease. But to me, reacting meant getting angry, pushing for a cure for AIDS in our lifetime. Getting our lives back to normal.

Arlene listed on an easel the twelve most frequent "helping attempts" that often do just the opposite and become roadblocks.

1. *Ordering, commanding*
2. *Warning, threatening*
3. *Moralizing, preaching*
4. *Advising, giving solutions*
5. *Persuading with logic, arguing*
6. *Judging, criticizing, blaming*
7. *Praising or agreeing*
8. *Name calling, ridiculing*
9. *Analyzing, diagnosing*
10. *Reassuring, sympathetic*
11. *Probing, questioning*
12. *Diverting, sarcasm, withdrawal*

Am I guilty of any of these? Ordering, commanding? Possibly. Could I tone down my ordering? It would be difficult. I was always in supervisory roles in the workforce and consequently "in charge" of the home operations. Ordering and commanding were my ways of maintaining these positions. Or were they?

As I looked over the list of the remaining eleven attempts, Arlene's voice saved me from further self-evaluation.

"Before we break, let's practice some listening skills." *Arlene herself is pretty adept at ordering and commanding.* "Pair off, and one person will spend three minutes telling the other about an event that happened today. After three minutes, reverse roles so the listener then becomes the speaker. Remember, in whichever role you find yourself, be present and respond."

Adelle, a therapist, approached me for the pairing. For three minutes, I listened to her in a new way. I listened to what she had to say and responded in a way I believed to be meaningful. Then for three minutes I told Adelle about Gil's decision that very afternoon to cease taking the drug combination of AZT and ddC, a combination responsible for the probably irreversible neuropathy and painful nerve damage he was experiencing in his feet. Morphine would be Gil's choice for a replacement drug rather than the ineffective "AIDS combating drugs." Gil no longer wanted to harm his body with those experimental drug combinations. Palliative was now the keyword for his medical direction. How did I feel about his decision? I was in agreement; palliative care was hospice philosophy.

Did I really get all this information out to Adelle in three short minutes?

After the break, our group discussion shifted to Advance Directives and legal issues. I was familiar with all these documents: Durable Power of Attorney for Health Care, Power of Attorney, Living Will, and Last Will and Testament.

Gil and I had drawn our Last Will and Testaments B.A. (Before AIDS), when purchasing our home in 1989, eighteen months prior to the diagnosis. We then made an appointment with our lawyer to have the other appropriate documents executed A.A. (After AIDS), when disease entered our world.

A Living Will directed that no life-sustaining procedures, including artificial nutrition or hydration, be taken when either of us was unable to actively participate in the decision-making process. We agreed on this.

A Durable Power of Attorney for Health Care named each other as the person to act on the signer's behalf to make medical decisions upon either of us becoming incapacitated. We believed in this.

A Power of Attorney provided that each of us may transact business for the other, not to be affected by the subsequent disability or incompetence of the other. We trusted each other.

"It's important to discuss these documents with your family so that everyone is aware of your wishes," Arlene instructed. "These Advance Directives can spare your family members from making tough decisions during emotional times."

Gil had made copies of all these documents. He shared them with his mother. However, he never told me her reactions to them. I had placed my copies in the safe deposit box, not yet wanting to upset my parents with our world A.A.

"Your homework assignment: First, think about whether you should execute some of these discussed legal documents, although you may not be in a life-threatening situation." *We're one step ahead of you, Arlene.* "And second, practice your listening skills by letting someone talk for twenty uninterrupted minutes on any topic they choose. Be present, and respond only with eye contact and body language, no verbal communication on your part."

I was napping on the couch when the front door's closing woke me.

"So, what did you learn in training tonight?" His usual opening.

"Legal issues," I answered.

"We've got that all taken care of, right?"

"I think so." *Especially if you've gone over it with your mother.*

"It's been two years since we saw our lawyer. Could we make an appointment with her so that I clearly know everything is taken care of? I want to make sure you'll be okay when I'm gone, not lose the house and all."

"We can do that." I hated talk with such finality to it, but I knew it was necessary.

"Is that all you talked about? Must have been a pretty dry night."

"Listening skills."

Gil began to giggle. "You, listen?"

"Yes. And this is the homework assignment. I need to let you talk for twenty uninterrupted minutes —"

He interrupted me with a rash of tittering.

"Let me finish. This is a perfect example of the assignment. As I was saying, twenty uninterrupted minutes on any topic you choose."

"You mean to say you can't say a word while I'm talking?" He loved every minute of this.

"I can respond with pretty direct eye contact and body language."

"I know you can't do it," he challenged me.

"Just try me. Go get that egg timer." I was ready for the challenge.

For twenty minutes, I was outwardly silent and present. However, internal questions were formulating.

Gil spoke for twenty minutes, attempting to shield me.

"I want to talk about my mother." *Your mother?*

"I'm troubled by how I expect her to behave after I die." *What are you trying to tell me?*

"She'll come into our home after I'm gone and clear it out, claiming everything as hers." *What are you saying, Gil? Nothing here belongs to her.*

"I don't want you to have to go through this with her." *And I don't want to go through it with her.*

"I've spoken with my mother about it. I told her I would haunt her for the rest of her life if she even tried such a thing. Tomorrow we need to call the security company and have our home equipped with an alarm system. I'm serious about this. I didn't want to have to tell you this, and you probably don't believe me." *Gil, you're frightening me.*

"This has been heavy on my mind for the past year, and I need to be assured you'll be okay. Safe from her." *Can I ever be safe from her?*

"Promise me you'll call tomorrow so that I'll feel some peace." *How can I ever feel at peace knowing this about your mother?*

For twenty minutes, all I was allowed to do was respond to Gil with my eyes and body. All I did was nod.

See Appendix F: End-of-Life Coaching Exercise...
BEING PRESENT/LISTENING, page 249.

The Coma

One Week in March 1996

Gil sat perched on the edge of the hospital bed set up in the living room, on the evening of the coma, clutching his little black stuffed "Hug Me" bear. He was apathetically awaiting dinner. This emotion was a strange turnaround for someone who had found so much joy in cooking. His credo had always been: "Cooking is an act of love."

My "act of love" that night was a beef stew I barely found time to prepare and pour into a Crock-Pot to simmer all day, while I dived into the intensity of just being there for Gil.

From the rectangular cutout in the wall that looked out from the galley kitchen into the combined dining and living rooms, I scanned our reduced living space. This one-floor-level world consisted of kitchen, bathroom, and dining/living room with hospital bed placed center stage. At the foot of the bed stood his ever-tuned television. Gil was seated on the bed, absently watching it. I was sure he had no clue what he was viewing; it had just become a twenty-four-hour-a-day diversion, as he slowly retreated from the world of the living. News and weather channels were no longer important in Gil's world. Soap operas, vintage situation comedies, and *Oprah* or *Live with Regis and Kathie Lee* were the stopping points on his remote-control channel surfs. As I walked into the room announcing, "Dinner's ready, Gil," was I hearing the laugh track from some situation comedy he had probably seen hundreds of times during his forty-one years?

Did I detect the trace of a smile on his lips, before I saw his body suddenly go rigid and fall back onto the bed with his arms wildly thrashing, eyes rolling toward the back of his head? Was my dinner announcement the last words he heard from my lips? Who can know?

I dropped the two Fiesta bowls of stew, slopping their contents on the linen tablecloth, and rushed to the bed, enveloping him in my arms. I tried to calm and soothe the violence of his body with a mantra: "Gil, I love you so much. If it's time for you to go, I give you my permission to leave. Honey, you're going to a better place where there's no pain. You'll live on in my heart forever. Gil, you don't need to worry about me; I'll be okay. I love you."

I'd like to believe these phrases were the last words Gil heard before slipping into a coma.

I had yet to experience a death firsthand, but this was not the scenario that had run through my mind over the past four years. This was not the peaceful passage I was expecting. His body calmed so that I could reach for the cordless telephone to place a call to the hospice nurse, Norma. I lay holding Gil for the ten minutes it took Norma to arrive, ten minutes that seemed to be ten hours. I talked constantly to Gil, hoping and expecting to elicit a response from him.

Norma's evaluation, along with her phone conversation with Gil's doctor, concluded that Gil had slipped into the coma due to a brain seizure.

"Norma, I just cannot do this by myself any more. Two hours of daily respite from hospice is not enough." My plea was not just for myself, drained physically, mentally, and now emotionally; it was more for Gil, who would now likely require a catheter, oxygen, and body shifting every few hours to prevent bedsores. These were the things I was no longer able to do alone.

Norma assured me I had been doing a wonderful job, but now was the time for increased coverage.

Hospice aides started immediately and continued throughout the week. Now I was able to spend my time exclusively at Gil's bedside, sharing with him all the magical things we had done together over the past eight years. I realized my final words to Gil were neither the announcement that stew was about to be served nor my ranting of all the reassuring things I thought Gil needed to hear. My last words consisted of everything that was said and done during his last week in the coma. I had signs from Gil to confirm this belief. Out of each twenty-four-hour day during that week, there was one brief moment in which he communicated to me through eye contact, body movement, or attempted speech.

Day One

It had been fifteen hours since the seizure. Gil's gray, part-tiger and part-Maine Coon cat, Fiesta, sensed something wrong. It was the first day Gil had not reminded me to put ice cubes into Fiesta's water dish. The cat must have jumped onto the hospital bed, reminding Gil I was not doing my job. Fiesta planted himself at Gil's side and stared at him with those yellow, ancient eyes cat seem to possess. I saw Gil's vacant eyes move to meet those of Fiesta. Gil's hand rose, with an effort to make contact, but hand and fur did not meet. I thought I heard Gil mouth the words "ice cube."

Day Two

Father Dan from the local Roman Catholic church arrived at our door to perform the *Sacrament of the Sick*. Gil had been motionless for hours prior to the priest's arrival, but during the priest's administration of rites I could see Gil's half-lidded, glazed eyes move in the direction of the priest's face, acknowledging his spiritual presence.

Day Three

My mother came to visit. She sat bedside talking to Gil, lovingly stroking his hand. It was when she said, "Gil, we love you as our son," that Gil raised himself on both elbows. He stared intently into my mother's eyes for a brief moment, before lowering himself back to his motionless, prone position.

Day Four

I was smoothing Gil's wispy hair and telling him how brave he had been throughout the whole time of his illness. As I voiced how proud I was of him, I saw his eyes move in my direction, and his lips parted, as though he was about to speak. I lowered my ear to his mouth to hear him slowly and feebly pronounce three words, "You are brave." He resumed his immobile position, with no further eye contact.

Day Five

The television had been on constantly for four days of the coma, just the same as for the entire preceding month. Because neither Gil nor anyone else was watching it, I decided it was time to turn off the television and replace it with soothing music that might help Gil with his transition. I felt we should do one last channel surf together. I placed the remote control in his hand, positioned his thumb on the up-arrow button, and gently enveloped his frail hand with mine.

Stations slowly changed as we did the complete cycle of sixty-odd choices before repeating the rotation. It was when the station showing the soap opera *Days of Our Lives* appeared that his thumb slid off the remote control, and his eyes focused on the television at the foot of the bed. I found myself lying by his side for one hour, watching him watch television, wanting to ask him about these television characters so familiar to him, wanting to ask him about what direction their lives were moving, desperately needing to ask him what direction our lives were moving.

At the open-ended conclusion of the program, I silenced the television for the remainder of Gil's days.

Day Six

One last forceful mouthing came from Gil's lips: "Andrew."

"Yes, I'm here, Gil." The urgency of his voice startled me. But no further vocal response came from him as I sat on the edge of the bed caressing his arm, hoping for more from his lips. Both arms suddenly raised perpendicular to his lifeless body; his left hand met his right at arm's length above his heart. The left hand mechanically located the third finger on his right hand and gently removed the gold band he had worn on his finger these past eight years. This ring was one of two exchanged as a commitment of our relationship, a private acknowledgement of our union. His left hand offered me the ring as he stared intently into my eyes. I immediately took the ring from the hand of his outstretched arm, then watched as his arms flopped back, lifeless, to each side of his body.

"Gil, I'll always keep this ring close to the one you gave me eight years ago," I said, as I absently slipped the offered ring onto the smallest finger of my right hand. "They were always meant to be together, just as we are."

I stroked his cheek; the two rings on my hand clinked as they caressed each other. I felt wetness on my fingertips, and I noticed the small tear that had formed in his left eye, rolling down his unshaven cheek. Gil knew it was finally time to say goodbye to me. Returning his ring was his way of communicating this to me.

He died just hours later.

The gold rings remain together. They clinked on my right hand for two weeks before being transferred to a rawhide strand around my neck, where they musically chimed, hanging close to my heart. These two rings circled my neck for two months, before being hung around the little stuffed black "Hug Me" bear Gil had clung so tightly to his chest until the coma robbed him from me. They still create their music when I clutch the "Hug Me" bear to my heart.

Music-Thanatology

The Coma Week, March 1996

It was the beginning of the fifth day into the coma; I knew I needed a more peaceful setting than what was being offered by the television blathering away.

The compact disk player would accept six disks in its cartridge. From our diverse collection of CDs, I narrowed the choice of music to one artist, Joni Mitchell. I chose *Joni Mitchell, Court and Spark, Turbulent Indigo, For the Roses, Blue,* and *Clouds.* I felt all six selections were a good representation of Joni's career and mileposts of the years Gil had enjoyed her music. I set the random-play button on the remote control so that the eras of her music would be mixed. Consequently, Joni Mitchell transformed the tenor of our death vigil into one of peacefulness. At the end of each six-hour music play, I unconsciously repeated the CDs, in haphazard order, again and again, for a total of eight sets. For two days and nights, Joni Mitchell filled our living room.

Upon returning home from the challenging, official farewell trip to visit Gil's family in Florida, Gil had turned on all three televisions in our home, and at least one light in every room. They blared and glowed continuously for the twenty-four hours of each of his last – conscious – twenty-four days.

While he was still mobile, Gil wandered about the house picking up the corresponding television remote controls, changing stations and adjusting volumes of all three televisions spanning all three levels of the house. No two televisions were ever tuned to the same station simultaneously. I could walk from one level of the house to the next and hear snippets of The Weather Channel from the guest bedroom, *The Young and the Restless* from the kitchen, and an *I Love Lucy* rerun from the basement den.

In which room would Gil be watching what show? None. He usually could be found in a room with no television. He had recently lost interest in the outside world and its storms. He no longer lived vicariously through the lives of soap opera characters, and he finally had enough of the 1950s sitcom he must have seen at least a hundred times before. More likely, Gil would be found in the living room perusing the newspaper for supermarket coupons he would diligently clip and organize in his coupon folder. Coupons he would never redeem.

Television viewing was one facet of life in which Gil and I differed. I could probably live my life without a television. My total weekly viewing amounted to a half-hour each of *Victory Garden* and *Martha Stewart Living;* an hour of *Dynasty* back in the '80s, since substituted with *Melrose Place* in the '90s; and possibly an hour of *Masterpiece Theater,* a documentary, or a movie. No more than three hours maximum of television a week for me. I would turn on the set just prior to the selected show and immediately shut it off at its conclusion.

In the absence of a stable family environment, Gil was brought up with the television as a substitute playmate/babysitter. During childhood, he adopted television as his familiar, guaranteed companion. Through his adolescence, it became the nonjudgmental surrogate family, more easily accessed than his actual family. Television was always there for him. By the time he reached adulthood, television had become merely a habit. He barely paid attention to what was on, constantly clicking the channel changer and momentarily lingering wherever it stopped before moving on to the next station.

Our house resonated with the three out-of-sync televisions. As Gil's mind retreated and his body weakened, he spent most of his time in the living room, confined to the first floor of the house. To accommodate his entertainment needs, I brought the television from the second-floor guestroom and installed it on a chest at the foot of his hospital bed. This action broke my rule of no televisions in living rooms or master bedrooms. To me, those are the two rooms in a home that should be for the intimacies of voice or body, with no distractions.

However, my priorities now were to make Gil as comfortable as possible during what time he had left. The six-inch kitchen television, the only one on our first floor, was too small for Gil in his newly confined world. For the following two weeks, only the recently installed television in the living room would be on its twenty-four hour vigil; during this short span of time, only the lights on the first-floor rooms now burned around the clock.

Gil refused to voluntarily close his eyes. He told me if he allowed himself to succumb to sleep, he was afraid he would never wake again. So, beginning with the recent trip to Florida, inside and outside his mother's mobile home throughout the days and nights of that month-long visit he denied himself a restful, reclining position and fought slumber in a multitude of sitting positions.

I protectively had joined Gil in wandering the hours of darkness in the confinement of his family's small trailer, the claustrophobic yard, and the maze of mobile park roads bearing the names of tropical flowers. Ultimately, our walks would end in front of the television in the mobile home. That electronic appliance was his family. We all sat like zombies in front of the box that substituted for family conversations that should have been happening.

Now that we were back home, two remotes in our home living room controlled the one television. Gil used a fully functioning, universal replacement remote. However, I kept the half-functioning original remote tucked under a pillow on the couch. If I noted Gil dozing in a nearby chair, with my clandestine remote I would slightly lower the volume. The minute I decreased the volume, Gil would instinctively awaken, change the station, and thumb his remote to increase the volume.

With Gil days into a coma, I finally quieted the television at the foot of his bed with my semi-functioning remote control. I silenced the companion that had been present for Gil, not only during his lucid weeks of March, but throughout his lifetime. In the newfound quiet of the house, I selected the six Joni Mitchell CDs, playing randomly and consecutively for forty-eight hours.

I hoped playing music, which Gil loved, would be my way of offering an adjunct medication for his comfort. To me, the music transformed the death vigil into a tranquility that the chatter of the television could not match. Without the distraction of a television screen, the music allowed me to be completely present for Gil, meeting his physical and spiritual needs. I did not recognize what song was playing from which CD. I only acknowledged the music when the six hours had come to a conclusion and I absentmindedly shuffled the songs for another six hours of serenity. However, after two days of Joni Mitchell, the music became too familiar. I needed to choose music that would help Gil with his final journey, and the music that would provide comfort to those of us who sat around Gil's bed.

I selected six CDs to replace Joni Mitchell, music I felt would be meditative, inspirational, and possibly transitional. The array for Thursday's play was *Dream Spiral,* Hilary Stagg, electric harp; *Winds Across the Water,* White Eisenstein; Handel's *Water Music Suite;* and three Windam Hill Samplers: *Volume 2, 1993,* and *1995.* Again, whenever the music stopped, I gently touched the random play button repeatedly throughout the day and night.

The following morning, I left Gil's side long enough to choose six more CDs for the new day: *Reflections of Passion,* Yanni; *Garden City,* John Tesh; *Shadows and Light, Ambient Music from Another Time; Spirituals in Concert,* Battle and Norman; and Enya's *Watermark* and *Shepherd Moons.* During the middle of the night between Friday and Saturday, I ceased hitting the random play button. The living room became completely silent for the first time in weeks.

As I lay on the edge of Gil's bed, touching him reassuringly and speaking softly to him, I noticed his television remote control, untouched for days, on the aluminum hospital-supply bedside table. Gently placing his familiar-to-the-touch remote in his still, cool, right hand,

I enveloped this chill, which I did not yet want to acknowledge, with the warmth of my hand. I tentatively placed his thumb on the power button. The familiar sound of the television once again dominated the room as I moved his thumb to the channel up button. With slight pressure from my thumb on his, together we channel-surfed the television one last time.

The gamut of programming was immaterial as we slowly moved up the dial. Gil never paid attention to what was being shown and never lingered on one station for any length of time. I could see only the ever-changing blur of colors on the screen as we surfed. Looking away from the indistinguishable glow of the screen, I noticed Gil's half-lidded, glassy, dark brown eyes directed intently toward the screen. Could he see the television more clearly than I could? When the revolving stations returned to the starting position of channel two, we had come full circle. We cycled again until his thumb released the button on a certain program. We watched the show together to its conclusion, and then I helped him press the power button, returning the room to silence.

It would be a week after Gil's death before I turned on a television again. It took only minutes of CNN news to realize I preferred the peaceful stillness that had since entered our home. I did not feel compelled to know what had been going on in the world as I mourned. To break the silence, I would turn on the compact disk player and press the random play button, replaying the last set of music that helped both Gil, those around us, and me with his peaceful transition.

I have recently learned that making music part of the death vigil is an ancient practice known as music-thanatology. Its concept is that music can help make us fully aware of the complex needs of the dying person. The music may direct the dying person toward completion of his life, potentially providing a tranquil passage. There is thought to be a phase in death's process during which the dying person passes through a state of being neither-here-nor-there and no-longer-past-or-future. Being completely present for that person, and his or her process, is most important at this crucial time. Music is thought to be the centering for this continued presence. I believe music-thanatology worked for Gil and me. Replaying that chosen music reminds me of the peacefulness of the time Gil was dying.

"REACH OUT AND TOUCH"

Hospice Volunteer Training
Session Five:
Spirituality

October 11, 1993

"Yit-ga-dal v'yit-ka-dash sh'mei ra-ba..."

The words made no sense to me as the rabbi chanted the *Mourner's Kaddish* to our group. Foreign syllables I had never before heard spoken, yet melodious and soothing.

"We recall the loved ones whom death has recently taken from us... And we remember those who died at this season in years past, whom we have taken into our hearts with our own. The memories of all of them are with us; our griefs and sympathies are mingled. Loving God, we praise Your name."

The rabbi's presentation followed those of a Roman Catholic priest, a Methodist minister, and a Buddhist. So far, only the Buddhist perspective on spirituality during grief and loss had somewhat intrigued me.

However, the rabbi's views mesmerized me, as he intermingled English, Hebrew, and Aramaic words as though they were one language.

"*Kibud hamet* is the honor and respect due, even to a lifeless human being," stated the rabbi upon completing his introductory prayer. "And *nichum avelim* is concern for the mental, emotional, and spiritual well-being of mourners and the requirement of extending comfort to mourners."

His words made so much more sense to me than those of his three predecessors. Until the rabbi's presentation, the evening had been familiar, filled with talk of absolution of sins and conjectured afterlives. Much of the recited rhetoric reminded me of why I had left the Congregational Church decades ago.

"Let me share with you some of our ancient customs."

I was hooked. I had experienced Jewish rituals when I was thirteen years old; school friends were becoming *Bar Mitzvah,* and I had been invited to their services, but that seemed lifetimes ago.

"It's considered disrespectful to the deceased to be put on display in an open coffin," the rabbi continued.

Even my Protestant family adhered to this rule. I had never once seen a dead body in my thirty-six years. Three grandparents' funerals had been my only experience, with never a last look at the deceased. There was only a mind flash of the last time I saw them living or how I wanted to remember them from years past, conjured visions of staring at a modest casket surrounded by gladiolas.

"Burial should take place in the earth, as cremation is discouraged. And it must take place as soon as possible following death. The exception would be if the Sabbath or a holiday intervenes."

I do not know Gil's feelings on cremation, or where he would want services held, or even where he wants to be buried.

"*Chevra Kadisha* is an organized communal society that prepares the deceased for burial. It's an honor to be called upon to care for the deceased. If you are a part of this group, you also watch over the deceased and assist with the burial."

Could I spend such intimate time with a corpse?

"There's a proper way to express grief. Tearing a garment, especially nearest the heart is customary. This item of clothing is then worn for the period of Shiva, the first week of mourning, or even for the *shloshim*, the first thirty days of mourning. Again, the exception is the day of Sabbath."

This was a bit dramatic to me. And wearing the same torn shirt for anywhere from a week to thirty days?

"At the burial, mourners throw a handful of dirt on the coffin after it's placed in the grave."

That was a somewhat universal ritual. I had seen it done in movies along with surrendered flowers and other meaningful possessions, though our family had never done it.

"On subsequent visits to the grave, it's an old custom to leave a stone or rock on the marker. It's a symbol that someone has been there. Flowers are never placed on a grave."

A stone left in your place. I never did understand the need to plant flowers on a grave on Memorial Day weekend, to leave something that might die at the site of burial, unattended during the summer months.

I embraced most of what the rabbi had to say.

Arlene announced, "We'll take a break before analyzing our own individual spiritual needs."

The four clergy left, and I wondered if I would ever see this rabbi again.

"For a treat, there's no homework this week. Instead, I'm going to ask you twelve questions that I want you to answer with immediate written responses. Later, feel free to review and meditate on your replies. Ready?

"What is your concept of spirituality?"

A personal connection with a higher source that I have yet to discover. On the scale of one to ten, ten being highest, put me at level four of spirituality.

"Do you think there's meaning in life? And if so, what?"

Yes. A need to accomplish an important task within one's lifetime. If it doesn't happen, the soul will have another opportunity to "get it right" in another generation.

"What do you think happens to you after you die?"

The body no longer exists, but the soul remains – either at this level in another body or transcended to the highest level, never to inhabit another earthly body.

"Do you think it's necessary that people suffer before they die? After they die?"

No. But suffering may be the catalyst for the soul to perform its task. What I consider suffering may not be the same to another person.

"Do you feel you have spiritual needs?"

I don't know. But I'd like to explore Judaism at some point in my life.

"What do you do to meet your spiritual needs?"

Nothing I can think of.

"What do others do to meet your spiritual needs?"

I ask nothing of anyone.

"Do you believe God directs events on earth? If so, when and how?"

I like to think there is a "director" who's in charge of the plots of the movie of life. However, there's no control over the extemporaneous playing out of these scenes by the actors.

"Do you believe people are responsible for their illnesses?"

No. No. No. How can someone be responsible for something either inherited or acquired? People are responsible for their attitude toward their illnesses.

"Why is there suffering? Why do bad things happen?"

Awareness and degree of suffering are self-imposed. Life happens, both good and bad.

"Do you feel there's only one true religion?"

No. I don't believe there's any religion, just group rituals.

"Is there benefit in praying? If so, what?"

Don't people pray only when things are going wrong? Shouldn't praying be a form of self-meditation?

"Okay, that's it for tonight." Arlene dismissed us.

Once home, I had the usual remainder of the night to myself. No homework to complete. Rather than review and meditate, I chose to look at the course's suggested reading, *Final Gifts*. I was engrossed in the stories in chapter fifteen, "Choosing a Time: 'The Time is Right.'"

> *"Some dying people realize they will die more peacefully under certain conditions. Until those conditions are met, they may delay the timing of their deaths. This differs from knowing when they will die; some people do know and do indicate when death will happen, others actually choose the moment of death. Some wait to die until certain people arrive, or until others leave, or until the ones they care about most have the right kind of support."*

The sound of the door did not distract me from the collection of stories, but the resonant sound of Gil's voice did. "So, what did you learn in class tonight?"

"First get comfortable, I've got twelve spiritual questions to ask you."

———

See Appendix G: End-of-Life Coaching Exercise...
CULTURAL CONSIDERATIONS, page 250.

Nantucket

March 1996

"So, you guys had a good time in Nantucket?"

How could Sally, the hospice aide who has been coming into our home this past week for just two hours every day, know about that trip? Sally came to assist Gil with showering, dressing, and lunch preparation and to give him a body rub. What could she possibly have known of our visit to Nantucket? I did not want to have this conversation with Sally about that trip last October; I needed to escape to the store.

"Did we have a good time?" I responded as I headed out the door, shocked at her mentioning that island.

Each day when Sally was briefly there, I left the house for two hours to reconnect with life outside. I used this time to shop for Popsicles in every imaginable flavor. Gil loved Popsicles.

Blindly staring into the grocery freezer section at the many varieties of Popsicles, I remembered the seemingly endless ferry ride back from Nantucket to the mainland and the interminable drive back home to New Hampshire. Gil was a zombie. What had started as a day of frantic sightseeing over the entire island – by someone with an urgency to see it all – ended with Gil's inadvertent overdosing on medication. This resulted in a challenging return trip home in his state of confusion and unsteadiness. These horrors were what I remembered of that trip.

Home from the store, I unpacked various Popsicle flavors and noticed Sally standing by the partially closed bathroom door, allowing Gil a few minutes of privacy as he sat on the bath chair and showered.

I rearranged Popsicles in the freezer, and Sally continued the conversation she started earlier that morning.

"That's all we talk about every day." I wondered why this was such an important topic. Sally continued, "Gil tells me Nantucket is a beautiful place, and he has many stories of the wonderful times you both shared there." Sally listed them: our walking the historic, cobblestone streets downtown; the visit to Bartlett's Ocean View Farm where we bought fresh vegetables; Murray's Toggery Shop where I bought the Breton Red shirt I was wearing that day; Mitchell's Book Corner where Gil found a copy of *The Ghosts of Nantucket* for me to read aloud to him; and the weathered wooden bench in 'Sconset, where he sat for hours overlooking the ocean while I patiently strolled the beach, protectively within his sight. Sally reeled off these events she had come to know so well in her few hours spent with Gil.

"Oh, maybe we did have some fun on that trip." I tried hard to remember these events, misplaced somewhere in my mind.

I rummaged through a bureau drawer looking for some photographs Gil might have taken during that trip to refresh my memory of some of these possibly good times.

As I searched, I heard Sally announcing, "It's time for your medications, Gil." She assisted him in taking the rainbow assortment of pills that I routinely laid out four times daily on the bedside table. Three light-blue controlled-release MS Contin morphine sulfate, one white Bactrim, one two-tone mustard and yellow Axid, one pink Diflucan, three orange Klonopin, one blue Megace, one dark red Mycobutin, and at least one white immediate-release MSIR-morphine sulfate. This man who had had so much taken from him – career, permission to drive his automobile, and a lifetime of dreams – was no longer in charge of his medications; that privilege ended with his overdose during our trip to Nantucket.

"Look what I just came across in a drawer." I fanned them in front of Gil on the table during lunch. "Some photos from our trip to Nantucket five months ago." He showed no visible interest in the photos and immediately changed the topic of conversation to the flavor of Popsicles I found at the store today. Why would he spend so much time describing the beauty of Nantucket to Sally and let this seemingly important topic between us become overridden with talk of Popsicles? On he went. We talked of Creamsicles, Fudgesicles, and rainbow-colored Citrus Stix.

The talk of Popsicles continued during the next few final days that we were allowed to lunch together at the table. Popsicles were all he wanted to talk about. Why wouldn't he share with me his memories of Nantucket? Was he embarrassed by his unintentional overdose of medication that cut the trip unexpectedly short? Did he remember my anxiety over getting him safely back from the island and to the lab for blood tests to confirm whether the excess pills in his system were merely a mood elevator or a potentially lethal morphine overdose? Did he want to save me from recalling that chaotic return trip home by not talking about it, months later? That day, I could have talked calmly with Gil about that trip to Nantucket; but he avoided conversation of it, in favor of talk of Popsicles.

Days later, Gil could no longer join me at the table for lunch or even for our daily conversations of Popsicles. He no longer had the strength to rise from bed to walk the short distance to the bathroom. A portable commode arrived; it delayed the dreaded and anticipated catheter. As Sally and I attempted to move Gil the short distance from a seated position on the bed to use the commode, he resisted going in the direction we were gently leading him. Instead, he attempted with newfound strength to head toward the opposite corner of the room, pointing and declaring, "I'm going. I'm going now. I'm going to that beautiful place. I am going. It's so beautiful there. Now. I'm going. Now."

In response, I heard myself chanting, "Gil, I love you so much. You are so brave. You are going to a beautiful, better place. It's okay to let go. I will miss you so much. You have my permission to go. You'll live on in the hearts of all our friends. I'll be fine, don't worry about me." I spilled words I hoped gave him some strength to let go; but these words were voiced equally for my benefit.

As I chanted the phrases, Gil turned completely around and feebly pointed to the portable commode, "I need to go pee."

One week later, Sally no longer came to our home; her job ended early Saturday morning. I missed having her around for her recently expanded eight-hour shift, attending to Gil's needs during the coma, chatting with me when he was asleep. In her place, I had tea with Gil's therapist, Janice. She had spent time with Gil the past few months helping him work out family issues so that his remaining days could be spent with a clear, peaceful mind. Although I was unable to share it with Sally, I could recount to Janice the reality of that trip to Nantucket, of how Gil confused three orange Klonopin pills with three orange MS Contin morphine sulfate pills, doubling up on Klonopin.

I remembered the emergency phone call to his doctor, the urgent attempt to get him home as soon as possible via ferry and auto, the frantic visit to the lab to confirm the level of Klonopin in his bloodstream, the days of the drug's after-effects – drowsiness, dizziness, and unsteadiness – slowly wearing off. I told Janice how frightened I was by this experience, that those were my only memories of Nantucket.

Janice then began to share her Nantucket musings with me.

"Andrew, one day I asked Gil if he could describe what he thought the afterlife might be like, and he told me it would be a very cool place."

She had asked him, "Cool in what way, Gil? Cool as in 'wow' or cool as in temperature?"

His response, "You know, cool. Cool like Nantucket."

"And what makes Nantucket so cool, Gil?" She tried to find out just what he meant.

"Because Nantucket is a beautiful place," Gil said.

Her story intrigued me, and I shared the Nantucket photos with Janice. Unlike Gil, she took an immediate interest in them and remarked how well and happy Gil looked in the pictures. Here were the photos Gil took of me on those cobblestone streets, at that farm, and wearing that faded, pink Nantucket shirt. There was also a photo of Gil sitting on a bench at the beach, resting his weight against his cane. I suddenly remembered a beautiful day spent on Nantucket with Gil, and I was telling Janice the same wonderful Nantucket stories Gil must have told Sally.

I recalled the previous week's episode of Gil's pointing to the corner of the room and his declaring, "I'm going to that beautiful place," and I suddenly realized the connection Gil made between Nantucket and Heaven.

The Beads

Leanne, Sally, and I sat around the small adjustable bed. Leanne was our housekeeper and now part of our family of choice. She asked me, "Would you mind if I placed the rosary beads in his hands?"

Those rosary beads were foreign to me; they had been passed down in Gil's family of Italian-Mexican descent. They had just recently made an appearance, for the first time in our eight years together.

Another foreign object that appeared in our home only weeks before was the hospital bed, turning what was once a living room into a dying room. I noticed other strange objects in the room such as the oxygen machine, rhythmically and noisily in use; the cane; the walker; the wheelchair; and the commode, briefly needed but no longer in use.

"Andrew, would you mind if I placed the rosary beads in Gil's hands?" Leanne asked once again. Rosary beads were not a foreign object to her.

Leanne's voice returned me to our circle of three around the bed, and I finally said, "Please do it, Leanne. He would like that." I was sure they had brought him some comfort lately.

Gil never sought the comfort of the rosary beads in my presence. I would wake many times during the night to find them left in different rooms he had been wandering through these past few months of insomnia, nights of living the fear of falling asleep and not waking again, nights of "just looking at things one more time." I am sure he spent these night hours in contemplation. The daytime hours were left to surrender to brief naps, catching up on his decreasing need for sleep. When I saw Gil with the rosary beads and asked him about them, he would answer he was a "recovering Catholic." They were a way of reconnecting with the spirituality of his youth he had abandoned for the last twenty-five years. I could not ask him any more about the rosary beads; Gil was in a coma.

As Leanne carefully placed the rosary beads in Gil's still hands, resting on his stomach, the ringing telephone wrested me away from my thoughts about the spiritual purpose of rosary beads.

"Andrew, it's Ellie from Hospice." Sally, the third member of Gil's bedside circle, had answered the phone. Sally, by urgency, had also been welcomed into our family of choice. Ellie was the spiritual care counselor at hospice.

"Hi, Ellie." My voice betrayed resentment of the invasion of my remaining time and space with Gil.

"Andrew, I heard Gil has taken a turn. I want to offer my assistance to both of you."

"I'm glad you called." Some warmth began to flow. "I need to look into Last Rites." I did not know who to ask when that time actually came.

"What's offered now is termed 'The Sacrament of the Sick.'" Ellie informed me that it could be administered at any time during sickness or impending death. "Andrew, shall I make some calls for you?" Ellie knew we were not affiliated with any church or denomination.

"It needs to happen." I felt some relief.

I returned the phone to its cradle, and all three of us focused our attention on the rosary beads resting in Gil's hands. I watched how light from the sun reflected in the string of carefully arranged clear beads, projecting rainbows of colored light about our living room.

Leanne's voice brought me back. "Isn't it strange the phone should ring as I was placing the rosary beads in Gil's hands?"

Leanne shared this thought, and as she spoke the words "rosary beads," the phone rang once more.

"Andrew, it's Ellie again. Father Dan from St. Mark's Church is on his way over."

Panic set in as I relayed the message of the priest's impending arrival. I rambled questions to no one in particular:

"What do I give the priest for coming to do 'The Sacrament of the Sick?' We're not members of St. Mark's; he doesn't know who we are... Why would he make a special trip to see us? What if I offer a donation and it's not enough? Or maybe it would be inappropriate to give money directly to a priest... I've never seen a tip card listing recommended amounts to give priests for certain services..."

Leanne and Sally simply looked at me, no answers for my ravings. The doorbell rang, and I looked helplessly to Gil.

Staring intently at those rosary beads, I heard myself saying along with Father Dan the words of the Twenty-third Psalm. "Surely good-ness and mercy shall follow me all the days of my life, and I shall dwell in the house of the Lord forever." I had not spoken these words aloud for many years, and yet they flowed effortlessly. He asked me a little about Gil, whose eyes were focused intently upon the priest. Not only had Gil's brown eyes moved for the first time in days, but they also seemed brighter and wider. I told the priest a brief story about Gil. Father Dan appeared nonjudgmental of our home, of our lifestyle, of the disease. I followed his gaze, moving from the rosary beads to Gil's eyes. He declared, "So young." And the priest was gone as quickly as he arrived.

How long had I been mesmerized by one of the multicolored reflec-tions on the ceiling? During that indeterminate time, I recalled the many issues Gil and I had discussed in preparation for this moment. I then started thinking of questions Gil and I had not even thought to discuss. I pulled Sally aside into the kitchen to ask her how I should dress Gil when it was time to let him go, for cremation.

"Choose clothing he would enjoy wearing on a wonderful trip you two might plan to take," Sally answered, adding that I should select clothes I would like always to remember seeing Gil in.

A journey. I like that. "But Sally, there are too many of Gil's clothes in his closet to choose from." Panic set in again.

"Take your time selecting just the right clothes." She added that I should also pick out the outfit I wanted to be wearing when the time came for me to send Gil off on his journey. She made me realize I also needed to tend to myself.

One brief moment, again watching the rainbow on the ceiling, was long enough to see that Gil would love to be wearing those green plaid shorts, that red athletic T-shirt, the comfortably worn, blue, hooded sweatshirt and – what recently seemed to be always on his head – the plush, purple L.L. Bean baseball cap.

I gently removed the rosary beads from Gil's hands, and, feeling their angular texture in mine, I headed upstairs to our bedroom to locate not only this colorful outfit for Gil but also an assortment of summery clothes for myself. My choice of clothing was sure to defy the snow and bitter March wind outside.

Three O'Clock Chills

Upon arriving home to the frigid, March New Hampshire night, after spending four stress-filled weeks in Florida with his family, Gil immediately headed to the living room thermostat. He set it at eighty degrees, Fahrenheit. "I'm never going to be cold again," he declared. We had been wearing tropical shorts and brightly colored T-shirts for the previous four February weeks. I knew he was determined to continue wearing those same loose, comfortable shorts and T-shirts the rest of his time. I never once altered the setting on the thermostat for the entire month of March. Rather than adjust the room temperature, I gladly adapted to his balmy home environment by also wearing summer clothes.

During that month, a daily stream of friends visited; they came each time suspecting it might be their last visit with Gil. "It's like a sauna in here" was the usual exclamation, as they removed layers of winter coats, sweaters, scarves, hats, and gloves. Gil had no concept of the drastic temperature difference between the cold outside and the excessive heat inside. Our living room was a tropical world, just as Gil wanted it to be.

Two couches flanked the adjustable hospital bed that dominated the middle of the room. Gil would sit on the edge of the bed, tightly clutching his little black "Hug Me" bear, and our visitors would sink into the couches. They were upholstered with a fabric of peonies and raspberries. Had they been actual plants, they easily would have thrived in this greenhouse environment. A wicker rocking chair was also pulled bedside, the station for the ever-present hospice aide who would sit, unobtrusively, then disappear during these visits with our friends.

Evenings, I would catnap on the larger of the two couches. The hospice aides – Sally, Lisa, or Darlene – would remain bedside in the wicker rocker. Gil would sit upright on the edge of the hospital bed, holding his black bear and vacantly staring at the television. He was fighting the sleep from which he was afraid he would not awaken.

This became our daily, and nightly, routine until Gil had the seizure and plunged into a coma. However, this last week of March, Gil was in a prone position on the hospital bed, his black bear placed at his side. I was now the one who was afraid of the sleep from which he would not awake. Friends continued the visits by day; I continued to lie next to the bed by night. A rotation of aides continued the rhythm in the rocking chair twenty-four hours each day.

Norma, our hospice nurse who checked in each day, gently predicted that Gil would probably be with us for at least another forty-eight hours. She suggested I might want to consider going upstairs and trying to get a good night's sleep in the comfort of my bed. "Gil's and my bed," I corrected her. Lisa would be with Gil, and she would let me know if there were any changes. I had not slept upstairs in our bed but once since our return from Florida. We had slept together that first night home. It seemed so long ago. Because I had not slept much this month, the idea of stretching out on the queen-sized bed sounded inviting.

As I fell asleep upstairs, I could hear Lisa reading aloud to Gil. I could not make out what she read, but it was a comforting sound throughout the house. Hours later, my shivering body woke me. Why was I so cold? Did the furnace go out? I wrapped myself in a blanket and went downstairs to check the thermostat to see if it had been turned down or if the furnace had malfunctioned. It felt so cold in the house that I expected to see the vapor of my breath as I checked the temperature reading. It was set at eighty degrees, and the room temperature registered eighty-two degrees.

I walked over to check Gil, who was lying peacefully on the hospital bed, with Lisa catnapping in the rocker at his side. He was dressed, as usual, in just a T-shirt. A floral-patterned sheet, pulled just above his waist, concealed the catheter tubing and its receptacle. I touched his arm to detect the temperature of his skin. The area from his elbow down to his fingers was now as icy cold as I felt the temperature of the room to be. I pulled the sheet covering the lower half of his body up to his chin to keep him warm, and the room temperature suddenly elevated. The grandfather clock chimed three o'clock in the morning. Although I now find this occurrence to be somewhat eerie, at the time it did not seem at all out of the ordinary.

I knew from that moment on, I would not be far from Gil's side. Our close friend, Katrina, offered to stay with me along with the hospice aide. That night, Gil's last night, I took my usual position on the couch, Katrina, the smaller couch, and Lisa, the wicker rocker. Although the three of us would fall in and out of sleep that night, we all knew one of us would be tuned into our surroundings should there be a change in Gil's status.

I woke with a start and found myself involuntarily reaching for the comforter folded at the foot of the couch. It was chilly in the room. I wrapped the comforter around me, and I looked across to Katrina stretched out on the other couch. She had started the evening in the appropriate attire of gym shorts and T-shirt, yet now she wore full-length sweatpants and a long-sleeved sweatshirt. She was reaching for the comforter folded at the foot of her couch. Lisa, again napping in the rocker, had at some point during the evening gotten up and retrieved her insulated winter coat from the closet. It was placed over her body and pulled close to her chin. Gil was in his usual supine position, with the floral sheet covering both him and the little black bear.

I rose to once again check the thermostat for malfunction. As expected, it was set at eighty degrees, and the room registered its usual eighty-two degrees. This time, I did not want to touch Gil's skin. I intuitively knew its temperature would match the seemingly decreasing room temperature. I removed the comforter wrapped tightly around me and blanketed Gil with it. The room temperature instantly warmed, and the grandfather clock chimed three, just as it had done the previous night. The three of us, looking at Gil, said nothing to each other as we peeled off coats, comforters, and sweats in this house that once again felt tropical. Although Katrina, Lisa, and I had shared this three o'clock chill experience, we did not speak of it. It just seemed to be a natural occurrence.

The next time I was aware of the chiming of the grandfather clock was its three-quarter-hour Westminster Chime melody, the one that seems to go on and on and on. It was 6:45 in the morning. My head was resting on Gil's chest.

It was the clock's endless chiming melody that awakened me to feel the final, feeble pumping of blood through Gil's heart. That prompted me to hear Gil's last rattle of faint breath through his open mouth. That warned me of Gil's fetid smell all around me. That alerted me to taste my tears' salt, trickling on my lips. That forced me to see that a chapter in my life had come to an end. The grandfather clock had made me aware of everything around me. The grandfather clock made me face the reality that Gil had died.

It was hard for me to accept it, but I had no choice. I had just witnessed his death. Even though Gil no longer required my attention, there seemed to be so much I still needed to take care of – for Gil, and for myself.

My first full day without Gil eventually came to an end.

At midnight, I stared at our bed knowing that I needed sleep. I couldn't bring myself to climb into bed alone; I had slept in our bed only twice during the month of March, once with Gil and once alone, knowing he was downstairs safely watched over. Tonight, I was alone. I went downstairs and retrieved his black bear from the edge of the couch where I had spent so much time this past month. Grabbing the bear, I ran upstairs, avoiding the big, empty space in the center of the room where the hospital bed had commanded attention all month. The medical supply company had retrieved it earlier in the day, and I could not yet return the furniture to its usual position. Upstairs, pausing a moment again by the bed Gil and I had shared, I hugged the black bear and jumped onto the bed, pulling the sheet and comforter over my head and immediately falling asleep.

Intense shivering abruptly awakened me. I knew for a fact the thermostat was no longer set at eighty degrees; it was now at a more reasonable sixty-eight degrees. I shouldn't be cold. Alone in bed, I clutched the black bear to find warmth, and the grandfather clock informed me once again that it was three o'clock in the morning, my third consecutive morning awareness of the chimes. I got out of bed and went downstairs. I did not need to look at the thermostat to confirm its reading. I sat on the edge of the couch, staring at the void in the center of the room. A sudden warmth enveloped me.

The three o'clock chills came three consecutive nights; I have not experienced them since. Could it be that on those two nights before Gil died an unknown energy came at three o'clock to check on Gil's death progress? Its presence each time seems to have drained the house of all its warmth. Gil was not ready to go at the time of the first three o'clock visit. Was there a return of this energy the following morning, once again at three o'clock? Gil was ready; this second visit was three hours before he died. Was this presence there to assist his dying process? The third visit was during the night following his death, once again at three o'clock. And was this energy's presence for my benefit, to assure me Gil had successfully made his transition?

I do not know.

"DO YOU KNOW WHERE YOU'RE GOING TO?"

Hospice Volunteer Training
Session Six:
The Funeral Home

October 18, 1993

The table we volunteers-in-training circled was cold stainless steel; the concrete floor sloped to the circular, rust-stained drain. Walls of more stainless steel and surgical instruments of all sizes were reflected in the glaring fluorescent lighting overhead. We were in the autopsy room of the funeral home. I blindly stared at this table on which Gil might someday lie. I had to look away, but items in every direction reinforced death, images for which I was not prepared.

"After the blood has been drained from the body..."

Can I make it through this presentation? So far I had had no problem with the parlor. Its floral wallpaper, Victorian seating of mauve crushed velvet, soft lighting, soothing music – a room in which to mourn; and the showroom with its array of vaults, caskets, urns, and headstones – a room to conduct business. But this autopsy room, this was a room off-limits to family.

Yet, I was here. I needed to see this autopsy room, I just did not need to visualize Gil's naked, lifeless body exposed on the gleaming stainless steel, blood draining off the table onto the floor, AIDS-tainted blood washing down the drain. I closed my eyes. Nowhere in this room was safe.

The funeral director continued his presentation. "An autopsy is the medical examination of the body after death. Sometimes it's required by law; otherwise it may or may not be done according to the wishes of the family."

Gil must not have an invasive autopsy.

"An autopsy is done with care. Do not be alarmed that it might be disfiguring. The same holds true for organ donations."

Donation? Who would want Gil's diseased organs?

"Embalming is the chemical preparation of the body to prolong its preservation and appearance."

I would not want this invasive procedure. Would Gil?

"Cremation is the process of reducing a body to bone and ash through intense heat."

I heard Adelle ask, "If someone wants to be cremated, where do you do that?"

"Not here," replied the funeral director. "Cremations are performed at the crematorium twenty miles away."

Crematorium. To me, it sounds too much like "Holocaust."

"Arlene, could we also go to the crematory?" Adelle continued her questions.

"Yes. I think that would be enlightening. Anyone interested can meet tomorrow evening for a look at the cremation process."

Am I interested?

We then returned to where we started, the parlor, for the final discussion describing obituaries, burials, memorial services, and the prices of funeral goods and services. The director stressed thinking ahead, being informed, and making thoughtful decisions in advance, eliminating the added weight placed on a family during their grief.

I was on information overload. Is this why Arlene had initially told me that hospice training might not be appropriate for me? Maybe she was considering the stage of caregiving I was in. I needed to prove her initial determination wrong; I was strong. We were not going through a stage, or so I kept telling myself. Gil was outwardly healthy. There were no signs of illness. Yet.

"Good night, everyone," said Arlene. "This session was full of information. Anyone interested in going to the crematorium can meet here tomorrow night."

I came home to a flashing red light indicating Gil's voice on the answering machine. "Hi, Honey. There have been heavy winds and a lot of power outages, so I need to work an extra shift. They're putting us up in a hotel, so I'll see you tomorrow night. Love you." *Beep.*

———

The entire group turned out for the following evening's crematorium visit. This time, we were in a closed chamber with a massive flame outlet above our heads.

"The body is placed on this spot in a pressboard coffin." A different funeral director was giving us yet another tour of death. However, in this room, I could look away from the flame jet and see four bare walls and floor. "The flame shoots out and down from above and incinerates everything below to cremated remains. When cooled, these are carefully scooped and placed in a blue cardboard box, which is encased in a burgundy velvet sack."

Let me out of here. It's too claustrophobic.

"I'd like to show you what cremated remains look like. They really are not ashes as you know them."

They did not look like ashes at all. They were irregular shapes and small white bone fragments in the colors of black, gray, white, and rose.

"What are all those blue boxes over there?" Adelle, always full of questions, pointed to a large shelving unit in the next room.

"Those are remains yet to be claimed. Sometimes the family is not sure what to do with the cremated remains, so they leave them here until they know."

Or leave them here because they can't deal with them. How could anyone leave someone he loved on a shelving unit with boxes of other anonymous ashes?

"Okay, if there are no more questions, I'll see you next week." Arlene ended the evening with her usual buoyancy, in defiance of the two consecutive nights' subject matter.

"Wait one minute," she called to us as we filed out. "The homework is to write your own obituary and plan your own memorial service. Make it easy on your family. Tell them in advance what you want."

I took out the sheet of paper as soon as I got home and tried to think about writing my obituary, but all I could see was a stainless-steel table with flame jets above, although the two were separate entities. Hours later, I heard the door close.

"Hi, Honey. So, what did you do in class these two nights?"

"Wait just one minute. Forget class. I haven't seen you for days."

We hugged.

"I don't know if I can work any more of these extended shifts. It really did a number on me." I could see his visible fatigue.

"What do you mean?" I asked, knowing what he meant.

"For the first time, I didn't know if I was going to make it through my entire shift. I was so tired."

The reality of Gil's illness hit me. Yes, we were going through a stage, probably one of many. I could no longer deny it.

"But I don't want to talk about work anymore. Tell me about class."

"I've had two sessions since I last saw you, and you'll need to sit down for this one. I want to share some thoughts on how I'd like my obituary to read and ideas on my memorial service."

"Yours? Shouldn't we be doing mine?"

The Obituary

April 1, 1996

Gil's obituary appeared in the newspaper two days following his death. I remembered the night three years earlier, as we each wrote our own obituaries.

The hospice-training assignment was to write your own obituary. Immediately upon returning home from the crematorium field trip, I had scanned every obituary in every publication around the house: the local newspaper, *Foster's Daily Democrat;* the closest metro daily, *The Boston Globe;* and a national publication, *Newsweek.* For three hours, I immersed myself in the details of the abbreviated lives of strangers. I was merely researching an assignment.

In each life story, condensed into paragraphs, I scanned first for age and cause of death. I looked next for the ratio of those who died in the forty to over-forty years of age range, our peers. I searched for causes of death: cancer, organ diseases, accidents, old age, and AIDS. When I didn't find a reason for death, I jumped to the paragraph that suggested appropriate organizations for memorial contributions, hoping for the clue. Was it a heart or lung association, or an ambiguous charity such as a Visiting Nurse Association or a hospice? I critiqued each obituary for originality, personalization, and structure. I circled with a red pen the ones that made me take notice, the ones that exhibited life of their own.

My evening's research clarified the standard of how one's life was presented to the world, one final time. Could I improve upon this accepted format without being too radical? My musings were interrupted by the sound of Gil coming through the door, returning home from work. Could it be midnight, already? Had I been engrossed with studying obituaries for three hours? Should I conceal my research from Gil, or do my usual sharing with him? Would this premature discussion of death be inappropriate? Here he stood, wearily, before me, although still appearing healthy and working full time.

"Hi, Honey. So, what did you do in class these two nights?" These were his first words as he removed his leather jacket, revealing casual work attire. He placed on the table before me a plate of leftover, marinated chicken wings. The previous evening had been a potluck night at work. Gil took pride in the delectables he brought to those once-a-week work occasions.

I had no choice but to reveal what I had been doing intently. He knew I had made the decision to participate in this hospice training course as a way for me to be prepared for whatever, whenever.

He grilled me each Monday night after training sessions. "There must've been something that's been holding your interest." Some evenings I imagined a hot, white light pointed at me during his weekly interrogations. Was he jealous that I was learning so much about death and dying? I found his weekly questioning sessions not antagonistic, but rather more urgent probings for immediate answers.

"Well, if you think writing your own obituary sounds interesting..." I offered the work of this major task with an open-ended, fill-in-the-blank void.

He answered without missing a beat. "Shouldn't we be doing mine? Give me some paper and a pen." He had a sudden burst of energy, after a day's work that had unexpectedly extended into two, plus the hour commute home. "I want to write mine while you do yours." He said that he would love to have the final commentary on his life because most obituaries were bland and usually written in haste, by grieving family members or by someone who didn't even know the person who died.

How does he know this? Has he been reading obituaries lately?

"I can guarantee that my obituary will be the exception," he exclaimed as he headed upstairs to first change his clothes.

As my training weeks progressed, I was amazed more and more that Gil wanted to participate in every detail of his impending death. *Should I be shielding him from such unpleasantness? Where do I draw the line of sharing? Or do I?* Gil interrupted my protective thoughts. He was out of his work clothes and now dressed in maroon-and-gray-plaid Calvin Klein boxer shorts and a black athletic shirt. We sat opposite each other at the dining room table, silently writing and munching on his leftover chicken wings.

The most difficult obstacle in this assignment came when I tried to identify the actual date and cause of my death. Superstition dictated that whatever is put in writing is sure to come true. So, I chose a distant date and a painless old-age death during sleep. Once these elements were documented on paper, the rest of my obituary flowed. An hour later, Gil demanded, "Read yours first."

He listened intently as I read:

C. ANDREW MARTIN

C. Andrew Martin, 93, died of natural causes on his birthday, March 12, 2047, at his home.

Andrew was born in Portland, ME, on March 12, 1954; he was the son of Donald and Nathalie (Murphy) Martin.

He graduated from Deering High School, Portland, ME, in 1972 and was awarded a B.S. from the University of New Hampshire in 1975.

Andrew's careers spanned banking to retail management. He especially enjoyed employment at Middleton Inn on the grounds of Middleton Place, America's oldest landscaped gardens (1741) in Charleston, SC; and Tuttle's Red Barn, America's oldest family farm (1643) in Dover, NH.

An active volunteer of Strafford Hospice Care/Seacoast Hospice, he promoted the hospice philosophy and AIDS awareness as a hospice spokesperson.

His life companion, Gil V. Ornelas, predeceased Andrew.

A celebration of his life will be held March 20 on the first day of spring at The Chapel on the estate of Fuller Gardens, Rye, NH.

Should friends desire, in lieu of flowers, memorial remembrances may be made to Seacoast Hospice, Dover, NH.

And without comment Gil said, "Here's mine." I listened with curiosity as Gil read:

GIL V. ORNELAS

Gil V. Ornelas, forty-something, of 42 Bridle Path, The Paddock, died at his home on ? of an illness due to complications from Acquired Immune Deficiency Syndrome.

Gil was born in Wichita, Kansas, on June 20, 1954.

A graduate of Bishop Hogan High School (Kansas City) in 1972, Gil was employed as a customer service representative with Public Service Company of New Hampshire since 1987.

Cooking was an important part of his life, and friends and family will sadly miss his gourmet meals. His spirit is with us each holiday season with the exchange of Cards That Care, his idea for AIDS Awareness Greeting Cards.

Survivors include: his life companion and caregiver, C. Andrew Martin, his mother, a brother, a sister, aunts, uncles, cousins, and many loyal and caring friends.

Another brother predeceased him.

A celebration of his life will be held at a later date. In lieu of flowers, memorial contributions may be made to AIDS Response Seacoast, Portsmouth, NH, or Seacoast Hospice, Dover, NH.

Arrangements are under the direction of ? Funeral Home.

"I like my obituary much better than yours," Gil declared with conviction.

Shrugging off the finality of what we had just done, he added, "Mine has personality." He proceeded to inform me that my obituary needed more work. "Not just the facts. Give information readers can use to get a feel for who you were."

Who was I? Who am I, and why am I doing this? Writing my obituary should not share the same sense of immediacy Gil feels to complete his. I probably have a lifetime to perfect the wording in mine.

"I'm glad this has been taken care of," he stated matter-of-factly, and off to bed he marched. He was also informing me, over his shoulder, that it was well past my bedtime, as it was now three o'clock in the morning.

Looking back on that obituary-writing experience, which took place two and one-half years prior to Gil's death, I am glad it was an exercise we did together. Gil's obituary appeared in our local paper exactly as he wrote it. However, he made two editorial changes two weeks before his death. Gil added the word "peacefully" to the first line, so it read "died peacefully at his home." He also needed to change the address of his surviving mother and half-brother, from New Hampshire to Florida. Gil waited until the last moment to document this family shift in his obituary, hoping they would be there for him at the end. When he realized they would not, he edited this information with much sadness.

All I needed to do to complete his obituary after his death was to fill in the question marks: age, date of death, and name of funeral home. In Gil's words, this pre-planned experience was for me "one less thing to deal with. Whatever. Whenever."

Although I paid the newspaper a fee for printing Gil's obituary, the newspaper still had the right to edit my submission. Our local newspaper ran the obituary exactly as Gil wrote it, however, a more conservative New Hampshire newspaper, *The Manchester Union Leader,* chose to edit his submitted obituary in many ways, changing its entire tone. The newspaper editors deleted the word "peacefully," as though they could make the judgment call as to whether his death could have been peaceful. Also stricken was the entire paragraph referencing his cooking, which was one of his greatest loves in life and the detail that most personalized Gil's obituary. And, most upsetting to me, they rearranged the submitted order of survivors, replacing me as the first listed with his distanced family members.

Comparing our two obituaries, I will have to agree with Gil. Mine does need work. Soon would be a good time to update it so that it will, in turn, make it easier for whomever, wherever, whenever.

———◦◦◦———

See Appendix H:
End-of-Life Coaching Exercise...
OBITUARIES AND MEMORIAL SERVICES, page 250.

The Burgundy Velvet Sack

April 1996

A few days following Gil's death, I received the phone call from the funeral home informing me that Gil's remains were available for pick up. I had toured the funeral home, seen the autopsy table, visited the crematory, and scanned the unclaimed boxes. There was no mystery as to what Gil had been through since he last left our home. Nevertheless, I was anxious to have him home again, zealous to carry out his final wishes.

The funeral director presented me with the blanket I insisted they cover him with on that last trip, a certificate of cremation, and the burgundy velvet sack shrouding the square, blue cardboard box I knew what was inside: the physical remains of a man reduced to the contents of this small container. Gil was not to be left shelved with the boxes of the unclaimed dead.

I positioned the sack on the passenger seat. The sun, intensified through the windshield, warmed my precious cargo.

I was not ready to drive the three miles directly home. Rather, I headed to a high point on Back River Road that overlooks overgrown fields and the waters of Great Bay. It was April. Still winter. Gray sky, stark-white ground. The rigid structure of the trees without leaves opened the view to the gray water of the estuary.

I sat in our car for an hour, talking to the burgundy velvet sack. I reminisced of the many times we had stopped here to take in the tranquility on the way home from the doctor's office with updated news of the disease's onslaught. Or after visits from his family members, when some venting was in order. Or when just being home with a rigid schedule of medications was a reminder of things we needed to escape momentarily.

"Gil, do you remember the peregrine perched on that obelisk over there? He flew away when you tried to photograph him.

"Over there's the farmhouse and the tree farm. Do you recall trudging those fields one cold December afternoon looking for the perfect Christmas tree? They were all so pathetic." That was the year I bought the artificial tree, I remembered, acknowledging Gil had become too weak to help me cut one, drag it back to the car, bring it into the house, and get it standing perfectly straight in the cast-iron tree stand.

"Remember when the deer ran across the road over there on our way home one night?

"Gil, is this one of our favorite spots where you want your remains to be scattered?" Only an hour earlier the funeral director had provided me with all the logistics of broadcasting ashes. All I could remember now were his instructions to keep track of where I scattered and him saying that I would need to obtain permission to do so on private property.

"I'm not ready to let you go, Gil." We had been reunited for only an hour. "Let's go home."

Once home, I transferred the velvet sack to the spool bed, my grandmother's bed, in the dark blue painted room he called his "morning room." It has now become my mourning room. It was the guestroom; but Gil had been the most frequent "guest" there. The burgundy sack once again absorbed the warmth of the sun filtering through white, wooden-slatted shutters. Here in this room he would retire after I had gone to work for the day, or, as his health declined, for whatever decreasing period of time I left him alone. This was his television room. Friends would sit bedside in the green velvet, ornately carved Victorian chair, silently keeping him company in my absence as he retreated into the safe world of soaps, *Oprah,* or Regis and Kathie Lee. I felt the solar warmth on the burgundy sack – the same solar energy that must have heated him on this bed during his final months.

Eighteen pounds of cat took immediate interest in the foreign velvet sack, rubbing against it, purring, leaving a layer of tiger-striped hairs on its smooth, yet rough, material. Just as Fiesta must have done with Gil on this bed. He stopped rubbing and curled up against the sack, as if he knew it was his missing companion. I joined Fiesta on the bed and lay opposite him with the burgundy velvet sack between us – falling asleep in the quiet, dark blue, sun-warmed room, peacefully assured that Gil was home again.

A Celebration of Life

October 1993 / June 1996

The second part to the hospice training assignment, the same week as writing the obituary, was creating your memorial service. The weekend following the completion of our obituaries, I brought up the subject of funerals. Without hesitation, Gil answered me.

"I want a party. A celebration." Gil already knew exactly what he wanted. "No sad funeral, but a planned gathering of our friends on a happy occasion." It was as though he had already been thinking about it. "It needs to be outdoors, with food, maybe music. I know – do it on my birthday." He even thought about the scheduled date.

This conversation was a bit radical for me. Once again, Gil wanted to do the hospice exercise right along with me. I looked over notes for my remembrance service: a small stone chapel hugging the New Hampshire seacoast, nestled within a rose garden; minimal words spoken by a few chosen friends; and the planting by the mourners of a fragrant, June-blooming *magnolia virginiana*. In contrast, Gil's idea to plan a party as a funeral seemed – to me – outrageous. Attempting to put things into perspective, I pushed aside my personal observance jottings and focused on Gil's rapid-fire, emphatic statements. I had enrolled in this hospice training course not to become an active hospice volunteer at this time, but as preparation for Gil's final journey. I needed to know as much as I could about what might lie ahead for us. If he was voicing his opinions for his own celebration, then I needed to listen to him now, while he was willing and able to express his desires.

"Gil, what if you should die shortly after your birthday in June?" I was trying to think of obstacles that might interfere. "Would I need to wait almost a year to have this proposed celebration?"

"No problem. I love the summer, so why would I die during my favorite time of year?" He seemed to believe he'd have control over his season of death. "Summer is for *futzing* in our garden, for working on my tan, for taking quiet walks with you around the neighborhood on balmy evenings." It was true. Gil loved summer. "I know I'll die on a cold winter day." (And he was right.) He went on to tell me that his celebration must take place on a gorgeous summer day in June. "Let's have it at The Common in New Castle."

Many summer days and evenings, Gil and I had set up our portable beach chairs to overlook, for hours, the harbor, lighthouses, and sailboats off The Common. I agreed it could be a lovely spot to hold his memorial service. His excitement was becoming contagious.

"I love to picnic there with you," he continued. "That's one place where I'm allowed to forget I have this disease." He added that it would be a peaceful spot for the perfect celebration. "It's spacious enough for all our friends." His momentum increased. "Of course, there'll need to be food, and Motown music... Diana Ross and the Supremes."

"Gil, this is sounding fun. Any disco dancing?"

"Well, maybe I'm being a little irreverent." That voice inside his head began suggesting a more sedate affair. "So, what about a catered dinner at the York Harbor Inn instead?" The event had suddenly taken a 180-degree turn. "It could be dressy. Scrumptious hors d'œuvres, open bar, an angelic harpist in the background." He fell silent for a few reflective moments. "No, think about it. Who's this funeral for?" But I was not sure of the answer to his question. I initially thought it was for him.

"Gil, you're on a roll. Write it all down while I'm working on mine. Then we'll compare to see whose celebration is more meaningful."

Why couldn't I be equally as imaginative and have as much fun as Gil with this memorial assignment? Was the topic too unsettling to me? Wrestling with his words, *Who is this funeral for?*, made me realize that it was actually for me, and for our friends. Not for him.

Watching Gil intently working on his service, mostly deep in thought but sometimes smiling or laughing aloud, I reviewed my memorial service for final editing. It seemed bland compared to Gil's concept for a celebration. As much as I wanted to match his excitement, I couldn't. What troubled me the most about his potentially delayed service was how it might affect my process of grief and mourning, and how it might delay our friends' need for closure.

I remembered how he closed his obituary a few nights before. It was with the statement "A Celebration of his Life will be held at a later date." He knew this is what he wanted. But just how much "later" would be appropriate? Weeks? Months? Almost a year? As it turned out, a few months would be the time span between his March death and the

June Celebration of Life event.

———————

The Celebration of Life took place on his June 20 birthday – what would have been his forty-second – two and one-half months after his death. There was much I had to do in preparation during that short time. I gathered a mailing list of close to seventy of our friends.

I tracked down a photograph that had been taken of Gil two years prior – a picture of a healthy-looking Gil, although viral-infected. It was a summer candid, taken at the beach. He was dressed in a white athletic shirt, showcasing his nurtured, mahogany tan. Gold-tipped, tortoise-shell-frame, prescription sunglasses hung from his neck on a wide red Polo strap. I spent many evenings affixing this treasured photo to the inside of seventy cards – the AIDS awareness Heart of Gold cards Gil and I had designed two years before. The card pictured a red AIDS awareness ribbon adorning a golden box in the shape of a heart.

That card was one of four statement-making AIDS awareness greeting cards we had designed and marketed together during his final two years, as a means of raising funds for local hospice and AIDS organizations. It became our way of giving back to these supportive organizations; and, equally important, it was a way for Gil to express his need to promote AIDS awareness in a healthy, productive manner.

Below each photo of Gil, I attached the invitation and directions to Gil's Celebration of Life. Each evening for the week it took me to finish this love chore, I hand-addressed seventy envelopes. Alone and completely unconscious to this meaningful task contributing to my process of grieving, I affixed postage stamps bearing the image of an angel.

After completing and mailing the invitations, I planned the menu for the celebration. Because it was to be a birthday gathering, a friend baked and donated a huge, three-layer butter rum cake, ornately decorated in flowers and slivers of chocolate. To accompany it, forty pints of every available flavor of Ben & Jerry's ice cream seemed to be the logical choice. Paper plates and napkins in six colors of the rainbow and two bunches of helium balloons, also in the same color spectrum, became the party's unifying theme.

June 20, 1996

On the scheduled day for Gil's Celebration of Life at his chosen spot, The Common at New Castle, a public park, I knew I wanted to set up under the solitary, sheltered, open-to-the-air wooden structure that hugged the edge of the cliff. Under this wooden frame sat three oversized, weathered picnic tables – perfect for the food and selectively chosen memorabilia representing the years we had shared together. I had called the park's office a month before to reserve this space, only to be informed they did not take reservations. I had explained my need for this protected area, citing reasons of potential inclement weather and expected size of the gathering. Again, I was told reservations were not accepted.

I drove to The Common early in the morning, needing to be the first in line to enter at its opening. I was preoccupied with three major concerns: Would I be able to stake out my chosen spot and secure my fortress for the ensuing nine hours until the start time of the planned celebration? Would it rain on the celebration? Would his family make an appearance at the celebration?

I was the first to enter the park and, as if foreordained, had first claim to my chosen location. Spreading a blanket and attempting to inhabit the sheltered space intended for many, I continued to worry about the obvious unpredictability of both the weather and his family.

To pass the hours before the 6:00 p.m. arrival of our friends, I meticulously arranged three of Gil's colorful fabric tablecloths on the three picnic tables. A teal gingham checkerboard, an outrageously colored runway of multicolored stripes, and a rose floral print transformed the split, gray-weathered wood into a garden. I wondered if this discordant collection of cloths looked too much like a circus. No, they were the reflection of Gil's love of color and flashiness.

Not wanting to set up too soon, I retrieved Gil's rainbow-striped folding beach chair from the car's trunk. I sat and looked out over the harbor, just as Gil and I had done here many times over seven previous summers. It did not seem natural to set up just one chair, so I returned to the car for the accompanying beach chair and placed it next to the one already stationed. Although one chair was empty, the two belonged together. I recalled our strolls along the cliff, the gourmet picnics he packed for our outings, and the solar eclipse we witnessed. With a start, I was brought back from serene mental wanderings by the sound of two hundred schoolchildren noisily emerging from a line of yellow school buses. It was an end-of-the-school-year outing.

The children filed past me, oblivious to my solitary, seemingly greedy monopoly of the three oversized picnic tables. The teachers and chaperoning mothers, however, glared at me as they passed, knowing they would be sitting on blankets on the damp ground. The sound of frolicking children became a white-noise drone as I gazed through blurred eyes toward the harbor.

The sound of a car noisily backing onto the nearby jutting rocky promontory reaffirmed this spot was no longer a tranquil space. A formally dressed couple emerged from the car. The man held an umbrella against the threatening sky, the woman a bouquet of wildflowers. A second car soon appeared alongside the first, and from it disembarked a heavyset, gaudily dressed woman clutching a book. The trio walked to the outermost outcropping of ledge and stood in an unmoving, intimate triad for twenty minutes. The slender woman, garbed in a muted floral-print dress, then tossed her wildflowers out to sea. The man closed the umbrella. The couple kissed and reentered the car, and the lone figure rhythmically threw birdseed toward the retreating vehicle.

Shortly after both cars drove away, the schoolchildren simultaneously boarded the string of buses, which departed in an unending conga line. I was left once again in silence, as the sun emerged from behind the thinning cirrus clouds for the first time that day. As I sat on my striped beach chair, cycles of life had played before me. I had witnessed a new generation of two hundred lives yet to be lived, and I vicariously had attended the solitary commitment ceremony of two individuals, the promise of a life together. Both of these life events had been taken away from me: a future, and a longtime relationship, with Gil. Yet, the afternoon's events reassured me that life continues for those left behind.

It was three o'clock. I had a Celebration of Life to pull together, with just three remaining hours to do so.

On those colorfully draped picnic tables, I placed two terracotta planters containing sunny, pungent-scented marigolds, Gil's favorite. Between these pots were two books: one, a photo album; and the other, a brown corrugated-paper binder containing "Memories of Gil." People could spend time perusing the collection of photographs or reading the collection of memories already assembled in this binder. Maybe they would add their own musings to the book. I did not know what would transpire during the celebration. This "party" for a funeral was a new concept for me.

Promptly at six o'clock, the first "mourners" arrived bearing food. They came with cut flower bouquets, potted herbs, and stories of Gil to share. Without my direction, the celebration took on a life of its own. People clustered in reunions or in newly formed friendships. Gil was the thread that quilted them together for this one evening. The Celebration of Life became the party that Gil had two years prior envisioned it could be.

It was a gathering of all ethnicities, all ages, and all sexual preferences. Most present were healthy, although some were sick with AIDS, diabetes, cancer, multiple sclerosis, and other illnesses as yet unidentified to me. There were our neighbors, our co-workers both present and past, and our friends both close and drifted. People from all walks of life, interacting so easily with one another.

The communing at the celebration not only permitted grief to flow but also allowed much love to surge. That night was the first time my lifestyle and relationship with Gil had been validated in my parents' eyes. They no longer saw their only child as a social outcast, marginalized by his sexuality, but as a magnet, attracting like and opposite poles of caring people. No other event in my lifetime, I was convinced, could have made such a positive statement to my parents.

The darkening sky reflected the vibrant reds, oranges, peaches, and pinks of the setting sun, and I said my goodbyes to the departing grievers. Nearly everyone was gone. Our gathering time seemed so short; it was now nine o'clock.

I was once again alone at the park, as I waved goodbye to the last guest. I gathered and packed away everything but one photo of Gil and the two rainbow-colored bouquets of helium balloons, now combined. To its dangling strands of multi-colored ribbons, I attached Gil's photograph. At that moment, I remembered the one overlooked detail of the celebration. His missing request that had escaped my hours, days, weeks, and months of preplanning. The music. Motown. Diana Ross and The Supremes.

I released the rainbow-colored balloon bouquet with attached photo to the heavens, as I softly hummed a melody. The balloons distanced themselves farther from me and blended with the darkening sky of Joseph's Coat as my humming turned to singing. My singing grew louder and more resounding. I was alone belting out the refrain: "Someday, we'll be to-geeh-eh-eh-ther." My rainbow of balloons melded with the spectrum of the heavens as they became one over the harbor.

"LOVE IS HERE AND NOW
YOU'RE GONE"

Hospice Volunteer Training
Session Seven:
Grief

October 25, 1993

"'What ifs' and 'if onlys' are a universality of guilt and can be a major component of either anticipatory or survivor grief." This was Arlene's message during our seventh training session.

Am I experiencing anticipatory grief? Arlene's voice was tuned out by premature thoughts of grieving. *Am I beginning to disconnect from Gil, knowing he is dying? Am I even entertaining thoughts of possibly reconnecting with someone else once I am Gil's survivor? Or will I ever set myself up again for the potential of loss?*

Arlene's voice became a waterfall of words as she continued our discussion with the tasks of grief:

"First: Accept the reality of the loss. Talk about the death with others. Understand that it has occurred."

Will people allow me to talk about Gil after he is dead? Or will they mistakenly avoid such discussions thinking it would help me move on with life instead of wallowing in the past?

"Second: Experience the pain of grief. Allow and encourage the reality of the loss to run its course. Otherwise, it will surface at some later date."

How will I experience pain? Cry? Be angry?

"Third: Adjust to an environment in which the deceased is missing and take on those responsibilities no longer performed. Become aware of the roles that had been performed by the deceased."

Just what are Gil's roles? Cooking, clipping and organizing store coupons, brushing Fiesta, consciously enjoying life. Whereas my roles seem to be the more responsible: juggling our paychecks to meet the monthly bills, worrying about everything, anticipating Gil's death.

"Last: Withdraw emotional energy invested in the deceased and put it toward new relationships. Make new friends, develop new interests, and derive support from a loving community of family and friends. You'll find this investment will last the remainder of your life as a survivor."

Won't life change enough after Gil's death without introducing more alterations?

I listened intently as Arlene spoke. This topic of grief fascinated me while I mentally started to list the anticipatory "what ifs."

What if... I can't do this? ...I start resenting him? ...He starts feeling indignant toward me? ...He loses his mind? ...Goes into a coma? What if he has to be repeatedly hospitalized? What if he dies when I'm not there? Or exhales his last breath in my arms? What if a cure is discovered but it's too late for Gil? What if I lose the capacity to feel anything anymore, with anyone, including myself? What if...

Then I started recording the "if onlys."

If only... there was a cure. ...I was also sick. ...I didn't have to go through this. If only this whole thing were merely a reporting error of a laboratory result. If only...

"After the break, we're going to talk about some of the grief programs Seacoast Hospice offers volunteers and the family members of patients." Arlene's voice abruptly ended my lists with one last thought.

Grief. Such an intriguing aspect of hospice. My association with hospice need not end upon Gil's death.

Arlene continued her presentation after the short break. "We offer bereavement support groups in the spring and fall for adults, teens, and children. Our bereavement program also maintains contact with the family of the deceased with handwritten notes on the one-month, six-month, and one-year anniversaries of the death. This continuing communication reinforces to the survivors that hospice remains here for them."

Bereavement letters. That will be my volunteer function for hospice.

"And you need to know that a hospice volunteer need not have a one-on-one relationship with someone who is dying. There are clerical, public speaking, and fundraising opportunities that are equally important. And oftentimes, to avoid burnout, it's healthy for a volunteer to alternate among these duties."

Bereavement letters. Because Gil is my "pre-assigned hospice patient," I could stay at home with him as I write bereavement letters to others.

"Upon completion of hospice training, we ask you to commit four hours each week to volunteer duties."

That's sixteen hours each month. Only eight full days or nights each year. Bereavement letters would be the logical way for me to fulfill this obligation.

"For homework, think about your commitment to hospice upon graduation, which is only two weeks away."

———————

I was in bed when Gil returned home from work. He poked me and asked, "So, what did you guys talk about tonight?"

"Grief and bereavement," I murmured, half asleep.

"I grieve, you know." He spoke with deliberation.

"What?" Still disoriented from sleep.

"I feel we're somehow distancing ourselves, and I don't know who's responsible. It makes me sad."

"Gil, I'm feeling that I'm not able to do enough for you," I countered, immediately awake. "I don't want to be asking myself some day if only I had done this, not said that, what if..."

Those "if onlys" and "what ifs" are already invading our lives.

Gil started to list some regrets. "I know we have our condominium, but I feel sorry that we'll never have a house together, one that needs to be personalized, a house with a yard and a garden for you, a house with a huge kitchen for me...." Gil began to sob uncontrollably.

"I'm mad," I shouted at him. "Not at you, but angry that you're going to leave me." I pounded my fist into the pillow.

"I want to know you'll be okay after I'm gone."

"I need to know you'll be healthy right up to the end." I looked for reassurance he could not give.

"I wish my family was more accepting, more supporting...." His sobs turned to wails.

"If only this wasn't happening to us. Taking hospice training and becoming intimate with death isn't making this any easier for me, or for us." I un-balled my fist and reached for his hand.

Then Gil seemed to become composed. "But it's making it easier for me."

These words assured me this was true. We had been talking about things for seven weeks that we probably never would have discussed had I not been taking the weekly sessions and been challenged with the presented topics.

"Come to bed." I drummed the edge of the bed with staccato pats.

He crawled under the quilt, and we both cried into the night. Was Gil thinking along with me that "what if" we held each other so tightly we could squeeze and wring the virus out of his body? Was he also pondering "if only" there could be a simple way to make this whole thing go away, once and for all?

See Appendix I:
End-of-Life Coaching Exercise...
REGRETS, page 251.

The Canvas Bag

April 1996

It was time to empty the contents of the canvas tote bag. Navy blue with vertical stripes of forest green, mustard, and maroon. That bag went everywhere with Gil. It didn't matter whether it was an overnight visit with friends; a trip to the doctor; or shopping the drug, grocery, or outlet stores; he always had to have that canvas bag with him.

Why was it so important for him to have it at all times? It was some days after Gil's death before I could bring myself to investigate its contents. As I pulled out each item and displayed it on our dining room table, I pondered its importance to Gil.

In the bag were two paperback books, a camera, assorted personal health care items, a small lambskin pouch, a sports water bottle, snack bars, an angel pin, an angel greeting card, winter gear, and a wallet. The bag contained what Gil must have felt were most important to have handy at all times.

Gil was not a reader, yet there were two paperback books. One was

The HIV Drug Book, which is Project Inform's comprehensive guide to the most-used HIV/AIDS treatments. On our ride home from the every-other-week visit to Gil's doctor, he would diligently consult this reference book to check the side effects and interactions of the drugs his doctor prescribed. The other book was a well-worn copy of *Circle of Hope,* a collection of short stories about people with addictions living with HIV; his therapist, Janice, had given this book to him. Although he carried this book in the tote for the last six months of his life, I did not believe he ever read it in its entirety, always reading and re-reading non-sequential snippets from it. I wanted to return this book to Janice. She would enjoy having it back, knowing Gil constantly traveled with it and must have derived some comfort from it.

I picked up the camera case by its rainbow-striped carrying strap. A black plastic film cylinder was tucked into the elasticized section of the strap, stitched for that purpose. In the zippered case was the Canon camera I gave Gil for Christmas two years before, an easy-to-use, do-everything camera. Gil took it everywhere, so I have many photos documenting our last two years, strictly from his point of view. He delighted in photographing every moment. Opening the film canister, I was not surprised to find that there was not an extra roll of film ready to load into the camera. Instead, I found prescription drugs; a readily available stash of quick-release morphine to temporarily dull the pain of his illness, or of life, mixed with antacids, pneumonia preventers, antidepressants, and appetite stimulants.

I flushed the film container's contents down the toilet. I was tired of being responsible for all these medications. Until I came across this little horde, I thought the nurse had forever disposed of all his medications the morning he died. I flashed back to the last two years of sorting and counting hundreds of these pills, compartmentalizing them into that cumbersome weeklong pill box, breaking down each day into four separate pill-dispensing times: breakfast, lunch, dinner, bedtime. This canvas bag doubled as his traveling medicine cabinet.

On the tabletop, I sorted travel-sized Band-Aids, baby wipes, adult incontinence briefs, and a package of Kleenex tissues. I often reached into his bag to find Band-Aids as he picked at the scabs on his face and neck. The briefs and baby wipes were never needed, but they gave him the security of knowing he was prepared should a dreaded accident occur. The travel tissues were frequently used for dabbing at his ever-runny nose or watery eyes.

The small lambskin pouch contained a circular, metal rosary counter and its instructional pamphlet. Gil's rosary beads, which left the house with him on his final journey in the funeral coach, also must have been kept in this beige purse of religious ritual items. Unlike Gil, I found no comfort in these things, and I pushed them to the far side of the glass tabletop.

Between my palms, I rolled his insulated water bottle, imprinted with sand dollars, picked up from a vacation to Hilton Head Island. It was necessary to travel with water, an accompaniment to his numerous daily medications. Across from me, I replaced a drinking glass with the sport bottle at what was once Gil's place at the table. I also arranged the two strawberry-flavored Nutri-Grain bars on the persimmon-colored Fiesta dinner plate. Our table was still set for two, as if I were expecting him to join me for another meal.

Angels came into sharp focus on the tabletop. I picked up the small red AIDS awareness ribbon pin, purchased during intermission at the play *Angels in America*. The other angel was a get-well card he had received years ago from a co-worker. The card portrayed an abstract angel, an image that must have evoked enough mystery of the afterlife for him to want to carry this one particular card out of the hundreds sent to him over his last years.

His winter accessories were in front of me, not needed on this mild April day. I caressed his coordinating, multi-colored, polar-fleece scarf and hat and tiny, black, knit gloves adorned with a pattern of Mickey Mouse ears.

Saved for last, I opened the noisy Velcro closures of his red, fabric L.L. Bean wallet. Even after I rifled through everything else in his canvas bag, his wallet seemed the most personal item. Yet, I felt I must investigate its contents. In it were a small pocket of loose change, a two-dollar bill, and a white golf tee. Gil had never golfed or shown any interest in the sport, or any sport. Why would he carry a golf tee in his wallet? There were also four folded slips of paper from fortune cookies long ago consumed:

> *You have the ability to sense and know higher truth.*
> *You have a potential urge and the ability for accomplishment.*
> *Time is precious, but truth is more precious than time.*
> *Good health will be yours for a long time.*

Truth, accomplishment, time, health. I hoped Gil had found truth and experienced accomplishment in his brief time of failing health. In addition, in the wallet photo section, I found his driver's license, a laminated card indicating his funeral home of choice, and three photos. One picture was of the two of us flanking the Disney character Chip, in Oriental garb, taken at Epcot. Another was a rainbow-striped hot-air balloon he had photographed two summers ago in the field behind our house. The third was a photo of a complete arc rainbow, also shot in that same field. Were these comfort photos, chosen from the many he had taken over the years?

I looked at all these items displayed on the table before me. There was a common theme in the rainbow of the camera strap and colors in the photos of the air balloon and actual rainbow. My eyes moved to the red AIDS-awareness-ribbon angel pin Gil had worn proudly, acknowledging his disease. I pinned the red ribbon to the strap of the now-empty canvas bag. It was time to place all these items, except the camera, into a box to store away. In honor of Gil, I would start carrying this canvas bag with me. The first item placed into the canvas bag was his camera, and with it, from that day forward, I vowed to record my new life experiences.

A Time to Cast Away Stones,
and a Time to Gather Stones Together

April 1996 to April 1997

I had been gathering stones for a year. Each stone represents a time
and place of scattering Gil's cremated remains. After I filled two small,
salt-glazed pottery crocks – one for his mother and one for me – I
dispersed the remainder of his ashes in some of our favorite spots. Gil
believed this ritual would allow me to always feel a connectedness with
him each time I returned to these locations throughout the rest of my
life.

During Gil's final months, I occasionally asked where he would like
these scatterings to take place. His answer was always the same, "Wherever you want." So I chose the destinations, and every place I scattered
his ashes, I picked up a stone.

I had recently learned that it is a Jewish custom to place a stone on
the grave, or monument, when visiting the deceased. Although I had
not been religious for two decades, Judaic rituals intrigued me. Placing
a stone is a symbolic act to indicate that family and friends have not

forgotten the deceased. However, I have been doing the opposite. I have been removing a stone at each of the scattering sites, so far collecting nine stones from nine scatterings. Maybe, because there is no one gravesite for me to visit, this small pile of stones will become a collective grave marker.

Among this collection is a diamond-shaped, gray- and white-striated stone with a bisecting white band. The sharp points of this stone mimic the jagged cliffs of The Nubble in York, Maine, on which I found it. This was the first stone I unexpectedly acquired, from my first April scattering. I placed the stone in the pocket of my winter coat. Weeks later when I discovered it in my pocket, it reminded me of the evening I had placed it there. The Nubble is a scenic overlook where we would take friends visiting from out of town; and this was the spot where Gil and I would make the annual drive, on a frigid December evening, to view the holiday-lit outline of the lighthouse and outbuildings on the island of rocks. I intuitively knew this was a place Gil would want to be, where he could look over the eternity of the ocean and feel the power of the winds.

It was two weeks after his death when I let a handful of Gil's ashes loose to the winds blowing around me on that spot. He instantly disappeared in all directions. I looked down for a moment to find him and noticed this small, banded stone at my feet.

Another stone is New Hampshire granite, speckled in grays, blacks, and whites. Four weeks to the date and time following Gil's passing, I strolled the gardens of our home with another handful of Gil's ashes. Here were the perennial borders that together we had tilled, planted, and enjoyed. Life was beginning to reemerge in our late-April paradise. I sowed my handful of remains in an area where pastel-colored hyacinths were beginning to protrude from the recently thawed ground.

Other selected areas were the circle where the budded, thorny canes of roses stuck out from the earth and the spot where the sitting bench would soon be placed again, under the now-blooming star magnolia trees. These were Gil's favorite garden spots. These were locations in which I would soon be tilling, or sitting alone on the bench. The early morning air was still, and the ashes sifted from my hand, landing where I directed them around the tender shoots emerging from the earth. Looking at the empty spot where the bench would soon return for the season, I noticed a smooth, flat, oval granite stone. I picked it up and placed it in the pocket of the leather jacket I was wearing, Gil's jacket. Had there been a body of water nearby, this stone would have been suited perfectly for skipping across its surface.

The largest of the seven is a black stone from Newport, Rhode Island. I picked it up during a mid-May stroll along the historic Cliff Walk. To the right side of the Walk were mansions; to the left, the horizon defining the meeting of sea and sky. Anticipating my destination, I chanted the names of the houses as I passed: "The Elms, Chateau-sur-Mer, The Breakers, Rosecliff, Lady Astor's Beechwood."

Around a bend, I saw the verdigris of the ornamental roof belonging to Lady Vanderbilt's Chinese Teahouse, on the grounds of Marble House. Here, on a long-gone summer day, I walked the grounds with Gil on one of his "feeling good" days. Also here, on a cold December day when Gil could barely walk due to the pain of his neuropathy, we viewed the mansion's holiday decorations. This was another spot where Gil needed to be, where I needed him to be.

I let loose my handful of Gil's ashes, and they seemed to hang suspended for minutes before dissipating. It was a smooth, black stone that I picked up that day. I kept my hand in my pocket and held the rock tightly. The sun had heated its dark color and generated warmth to my hand for what seemed hours. Today, as I hold this black, oval stone, it no longer radiates the heat from that day. It makes me long for the heat that once emanated from it, and yearn for the warmth of holding Gil once again.

The amethyst-colored rock appeared brilliant when wet and now dulls when dry. Memorial Day took me to the Wentworth-Coolidge Mansion in Portsmouth, New Hampshire, where Gil and I would traditionally picnic, inhaling the fragrance of the state's oldest lilacs. I needed to be once again overwhelmed by that aroma. The lilacs were in full bloom. I walked to the water's edge and broadcast my handful of Gil's remains. The air was still, and the contents just sifted between my fingers, dusting the surface of the water below before disappearing. A vibrant, purple-colored, triangular stone marked their landing spot, and I reached into the shallow water to retrieve it. I clutched this stone, returning along a natural path of ancient, eternal lilacs. Today, holding this stone, I notice it no longer has its vibrant colorings of that day; but it has the power to conjure the events of that day and many other lilac-scented days past and future.

The egg-shaped, white quartz stone was given to me by a friend after the only group-witnessed scattering, the one that concluded our celebration of Gil's life at Great Island Common in New Castle, New Hampshire. An egg symbolizes birth; and the June memorial celebration was held on Gil's birthday. That Celebration of Life sunset scattering was probably the most dramatic of all. I let Gil's remains go with a broad sweep of my arm, and then I focused on the lighthouse in the sheltered harbor until tears blurred my vision. Someone, unidentified, lovingly placed in my hand this egg-shaped stone. I repeatedly squeezed the stone, coddled it in my pants pocket, and returned to the celebration of closure.

There is a small, gray- and white-mottled stone; it reminds me of that July day on Herring Cove Beach in Provincetown, Massachusetts. This was another place of good memories of my time with Gil. It was also a site of happiness for Gil and his friends before I entered his life. I felt the heat of the sun penetrate my body as I lay stretched on the teal- and white-striped, GVO-monogrammed towel, Gil's initials. My hands simultaneously smoothed the sand on either side of me until I came across this speckled stone. Its unexpected appearance between my fingers reminded me that I had something to do other than lie in the sun, staring at the cloudless sky, listening to the droning rhythm of the surf moving sand and stones in its receding wake.

I placed this stone in my backpack and retrieved a handful of Gil's ashes from the glass Mason jar. I walked to a point where the foamy, gray-green-colored water met the clean, damp beach sand. There is where I let him go. Ashes surrealistically swirled in a jetty around me on a windless day, then landed briefly on the calm surface of the ocean before commingling with froth. This was my most powerful, most spiritual scattering. I felt Gil's energy surround me for the first time since his death. The sun hid behind a large cloud and then reemerged, seemingly brighter. There was also a sudden enveloping, roaring sound, as though I had picked up two large seashells and placed them over my ears. The warm landward breeze seemed to spiral around me as though I were in the eye of a storm. I absorbed his presence for the longest time, resolving that no other scattering could match the peace and connectedness I felt there that day.

A brittle sandstone disintegrates in my hand as I hold it. It had been months between that last spiritual scattering in Provincetown and my next ritual on an October day, when I trekked the deserted beach in Ogunquit, Maine. Once again, this beach was a meaningful location for both Gil alone and for the two of us together. Miles down the beach a wooden footbridge spanned the endangered dunes, connecting the open ocean and beach to a protected inlet. The apex of the bridge gave me a view commanding all terrains: open, endless sea; sand and sky; tufted grasses; undulating dunes; and serene inlet. I let him go, and rather than watch the remains commingle with the sand and dune grass below, I looked upward at wispy, spiky cloud formations against the bluest sky. Through these clouds I saw the sun – the same sun under which Gil spent many hours here on this beach, perfecting his tan and socializing with his community of sun worshipers. On the footbridge, as I returned, I found the fragile, rust-stained, rectangular stone and placed it in my sweater pocket. This easily disintegrating sandstone that I now rub reminds me of this particular scattering and of our carefree days of sun and sand, now lost.

The most beautiful stone in my collection is a trapezoid. Its four sides outline alternating shimmering stripes of dark and light quartz and glints of mica. This stone comes from "that beautiful place," Nantucket, Massachusetts; this stone's origin makes it my most precious. I found it near the spot where Gil had once sat a year ago, overlooking the ocean for hours in deep contemplation. Only a year later, the remaining late-October winds from a retreating nor'easter tore the handful of Gil's ashes from my hand. They were deposited in a rippling pattern along the water's edge. I stood and watched as each encroaching wave came closer to the string of ashes, distinctively displayed on Siasconset Beach. The backdrop of fine, beige beach sand showcased the contrasting coarse particles of Gil's remains, in their grays and blacks and whites. Eventually, one wave obliterated all traces of the pattern. The receding wave accepted Gil's remains, leaving my most valued stone in its wake. A perfect, precious exchange. I picked it up and placed it lovingly in the same winter coat pocket in which I had placed the first stone the April before.

One more location remained to perform my last ceremonial scattering, and it would occur near the one-year anniversary of Gil's death. My collection of stones would then total eight. The now nearly empty, blue cardboard box, shrouded by the burgundy velvet bag, reminded me of my final scattering ritual. I visualized selecting one last stone amongst the numerous vacated seashells deposited on the beach at Edisto Island, South Carolina. This is the beach where Gil and I huddled, wrapped in a blanket, watching the most magnificent sunset we would ever enjoy together. This is where I knew I would find the stone that would reflect the warm colors of that sunset, as I returned the last of what remained of Gil to this earth.

After gathering this last precious stone, the time would come to cast away stones. I envisioned planting a tree and around its base placing the nine stones of various shapes, colors, textures, origins. And memories.

The *Yahrzeit* Candle

March 29-30, 1997

It was 7:30 on the night before Easter Sunday, and I was about to light my first *Yahrzeit* candle. Lev Baesh gave this memorial light to me. Two and one-half years after hearing one rabbi's spiritual presentation at a hospice training session, another rabbi intimately entered my world. It was this rabbi, my new life partner, who presented the candle to me so that I could observe the one-year anniversary of Gil's journey with this Jewish symbol of reverence. This candle-lighting custom began in Talmudic times, and, according to Jewish custom, the candle and its flame symbolize the essence of man. How appropriate that I would be lighting a candle for Gil, who, as his life waned, constantly had a votive candle burning at his side.

Rabbi Lev told me this candle would burn for at least twenty-four hours. I was to light it that night, at sunset, on the eve of the anniversary of Gil's death. Sunset, I'd learned, is the start of the next Jewish day. This candle would burn at my side all night into the next evening; and its flame would honor the anniversary date, or *Yahrzeit*, of Gil's death.

Although I was not Jewish, I found much comfort in lighting this white paraffin *Yahrzeit* candle. I placed the candle on the mahogany spinet piano in the living room and lit its wick, illuminating the darkening room.

It was now time to begin my personal "egg hunt" in preparation for the next day's "holiday." There would be no customary ham dinner served in my home that Easter Sunday. Mine would not be the traditional hunt for hidden, colored eggs. I had Gil's *Yahrzeit* to observe, with a newly discovered ritual from a religion that was not mine.

I wanted to locate the items I had displayed on the piano last year at this time. I attempted to resurrect the scene from last year: a cane; a framed photograph; an obituary article; sympathy cards; a memory book entitled "Gil Victor Ornelas: A Celebration of Life;" and his knitting needles, with an attached ball of multi-colored yarn.

I knew exactly where the adjustable, lightweight aluminum cane could be found. It had been leaning in the far corner of the guest bedroom, for lack of any more appropriate place. I removed the cane from its sheltered corner and tapped the floorboards with its cushioned tip, worn predominately on the right side. I had not realized, until then, how much I missed that rhythmic, punctuated tapping as Gil tested every surface.

This cane was originally intended as a Christmas gift from my parents to my grandmother; but ninety-five-year-old Nana, who died the summer before Gil, no longer had need for a cane at that end stage of her life. It therefore remained wrapped in candy cane-patterned gift paper in the closet at my parents' house. When Gil expressed an interest in acquiring a cane to steady his wobbles, my parents lovingly presented him with Nana's holiday-wrapped staff. Gil deftly removed the yards of coiled paper and immediately took the cane for a test walk. For as long as he was able to stroll, the cane never left his side. I found that the first recovered item on my scavenger hunt list leaned nicely against the support of the spinet.

I questioned locating the framed photograph of a young and handsome Gil, the one I displayed on the piano last year. Should I once again showcase a healthy image, or should I exhibit one that accurately reflected Gil a year earlier? It was time for me to confront those photos. I fished under the guestroom bed for a wanting-to-be-forgotten shoebox. My sweeping arm reluctantly located the second item of my hunt. Quickly flicking through the photos in the shoebox, I chose three that seemed to disturb me the least.

Who was this man in these photographs? Were these pictures from the 1940s of a forty-something man rescued from a death camp? Or were these pictures of a forty-one-year-old Gil, past the point of being rescued from his personal holocaust? The photos revealed a man so thin that bones protruded through sallow-colored skin. A wispy beard thinly veiled his drawn facial skin. Jaundiced eyes were sunken. Clothes hung loosely on his body as he gave the camera a vacant look in each picture. Why did I not see Gil this way in his final days? Was it his peace, and his will to live, that masked from me the disfigurement of his last months, his last days? I needed to display these photos on the piano this year to acknowledge the horror of his disease.

I looked away from the three photographs in an attempt to recall my mental Easter egg hunt list. The next item to locate was the obituary. I knew exactly where it was. I had tucked it away in my no-longer-read Bible in a bedside drawer. This Bible seemed to be the most logical place to keep the rectangular, laminated copy of the newspaper obituary article, presented to me by the funeral home along with the blue cardboard box of cremated remains. I found the obituary inserted in the *Book of Psalms.* I did not intentionally place it in this particular section of the Bible, and it did not mark any poignantly chosen verse. Yet, Gil's obituary in itself was a psalm, written in his own words.

On the piano last year sprawled a basket containing one hundred sympathy cards of various spiritual, religious, angelic, celestial, and floral scenes. These cards were nestled in a wicker breadbasket, hastily taken from the kitchen, its wicker spray-painted gold by Gil years ago. The cards were still in that basket, in a storage box in the attic. I decided to eliminate the basket of sympathy cards from last year's display on the piano. I felt no need to rummage through them, looking for past words of comfort. In their place this year, I would display the two cards I received this week, acknowledging this important anniversary date – Gil's *Yahrzeit.*

It seemed almost everyone's lives had gone on since that day a year ago. The one hundred people who had sent condolences had probably assumed my life had also gone on. Yet, two friends were acutely aware of the hurt and feelings of loss that still remained within me. Their two cards outweighed the hundred stored above in the dark, cold attic. I did not have to hunt for these two cards, as they were already in place on the piano, next to the burning *Yahrzeit* candle.

I noticed the candle had a quarter-inch layer of clear, melted paraffin floating above the yet unmelted, opaque-white wax below. Where was the time going?

My hunt continued for the "Celebration of Life" book, as the candle continued to burn. The past year, the scrapbook I displayed on the piano consisted only of the front and back brown, corrugated covers tied together with two leather strands. Within months, the book housed seventy-one pages of wonderful memories of Gil, written from many perspectives. I remembered where I had stored it. I removed the book from the sepulcher of the piano bench and placed it on the rack intended for sheet music. Maybe tonight I would read this book from beginning to end, something I had not yet been able to do.

The knitting needles were the last item in my search. Once they were located, I could rest. My homage to Gil would be complete. They must, I recalled, be in that cane-woven step basket. I found them at the bottom of the basket, buried by many hand-rolled balls of yarn. I held two blue, #10 aluminum knitting needles, attached to a ball of multi-colored yarn and connected to an unfinished dishcloth. Although those needles were silenced more than a year earlier, I could still hear their labored clicking and clacking as they once struck each other.

My mother taught Gil to knit these plain square absorbent dish-cloths for a mental distraction. She attempted to share different patterns and shapes, but Gil stuck to one simple creation. He achieved diversity by mixing and matching every available skein of colored yarn; no two cloths were ever alike. Remnants of leftover balls of yarn would eventually find a home in one cloth. Gil's incessant knitting occupied his hands, and mind, during the final years of his life. I debated having someone finish this last dishcloth; but as I placed it on the piano, I realized I needed to leave it just as it was: a reminder that we leave unfinished business behind when we die.

The midnight chiming of the grandfather clock reminded me I had spent four and one-half hours completing my hunt, displaying the items as though they were trophies. It was comforting to hear once again the melodies of the clock each quarter hour. I had silenced the clock a year ago; its three-quarter-hour measures immediately brought me back to that moment when Gil died. I reactivated the chiming mechanism earlier that evening, so I could awaken to the chimes playing their 6:45 aria the next morning, just as I heard them play a year past when Gil exhaled his last breath.

Realizing I felt weary, I removed two items from the piano. In one hand was the "Celebration of Life" scrapbook, and in the other the still-lit *Yahrzeit* candle. How many memory pages would I be able to read tonight before I allowed myself sleep, comforted by the memorial flame burning throughout the night? When I awoke in the morning to this still-illuminating Judaic flame, the *Yahrzeit* candle coincidentally burning on Easter Sunday would remind me that this new day would be my personally created ritual day of remembrance.

No Funeral, No Cemetery

June 1997

I was halfway up the steep slope and thankful for the sight of the small cemetery, situated in the woods on the edge of the road. It was a perfect place to stop and rest from the exhausting, late-afternoon bicycle ride that was testing my physical endurance. A quick rest amongst the rows of monuments was all I needed to reenergize and continue pedaling up the incline and through the lonely, meandering roads of Wakefield, New Hampshire. Why was I not in my room writing? I was at the Molasses Pond Summer Writers' Conference for the week; no phone, no television, and no interruptions. I should be writing under these perfect conditions. However, I was feeling a major interruption in my creative flow. Today would have been Gil's forty-third birthday, and I needed to clear my head with a grueling bicycle ride.

I sat on the granite stone that borders the cemetery. Droplets of perspiration, or tears, stung my eyes; my heart pumped wildly, breath punctuated in and out, and my mind was now allowed to wander to thoughts of Gil.

Can you remember me?

I don't want to forget you.

Do you miss me?

I'm so lonely today, missing you.

Where are you, Gil?

I'm struggling to find you.

Can you hear me?

I want to hear your voice just one more time.

Are you here with me in this cemetery?

You've got to be somewhere.

I'm still alive.

How do I keep you alive?

These were the questions I had kept at bay, replaced by the familiar rhythm of cycling.

I felt the need to sit *Shiva* once more, a desire to dredge up that comforting experience that had taken place more than a year before. I straddled the granite block, one of many horizontal slabs marking the four boundaries of the small cemetery. This stone would be my *Shiva* box for today; weathered, heaved out of alignment with its neighbors by countless winter frosts, and shrouded in gray-green lichen.

I was alone on this makeshift box, but I remembered a time when I was not in solitude, sitting *Shiva* in my own way. I recalled being exhausted and incredulous, at home for a week, following Gil's death. A deluge of mourners brought food and allowed me to share memories of Gil with them. This seven-day experience became my week of sitting *Shiva,* as described to me by Connie, a Jewish friend, during her visit a few days following Gil's death.

She told me *Shiva* was observed in the home of the deceased. After the loss of a loved one, Jews sometimes sat on boxes to show respect for the dead and to get closer to the ground, where bodies were traditionally placed. There was a *mitzvah,* or commandment, in Jewish tradition to comfort the mourner, to relieve the griever of the burden of intense loneliness. This was the concept of sitting *Shiva.* Connie continued by reinforcing that because Gil had lived here with me, his spirit was also still here. Everywhere around me could be found evidence of Gil's life work: a four-block quilted wall hanging over which he had labored, a collection of brightly colored Fiestaware to mask any darkness of his disease at our table, and the ever-changing holiday decorations Gil had proudly created and displayed. As she spoke, I mentally surveyed this "life work" and the nest – our home – Gil built as shelter from his illness. And from his pain. Yes, his spirit was everywhere.

Gil had requested no funeral. That week of being at home was the alternative – consoled by friends, expressing my feelings of loss. It was coincidental that I would be performing a ritual from Jewish religion.

However, this day there was no one in the cemetery to show me this *mitzvah* of kindness. Who would listen to me speak the language of bereavement anymore?

Did you know how exhausted I would be from the intensity of caring for you during your last week in a coma?

Is that why you requested no funeral or burial services?

You allowed me the opportunity to share weeklong grief last year in the comfort of our home.

Where are you today to give me the same permission to mourn?

Do I need a tranquil, reflective spot such as this cemetery to remember you?

If so, I do not have such a place.

From my seat, I surveyed this curious plot of land. Sharing one of its four granite walls was an equal-sized parcel of unused land, with its remaining three boundaries piled with gray fieldstones. An ancient field, once used for the cultivation of life, stood adjacent to this field, designated for the decomposition of lives. Within this pasture of the deceased were headstones bearing New England family names: Brewster, Wentworth, Hall, Milliken, Paul, Spencer, Wiggin, Sawyer, Nason. There was not one that matched Gil's surname, Ornelas. Here, in death, Gil's name would stand out, scattered amongst these Yankees, just as he was singled out in life by being both Hispanic and gay. I wanted to believe I did the right thing, for both of us, by following Gil's request for no funeral, the correct thing by scattering his remains in many of our favorite places.

Gil, where can I find you?

Gil once told me that he "wanted to be the sun, the sky, the moon, Disney World" – this during one vacation day, just three winters earlier, when we energetically strolled the Magic Kingdom before canes, walkers, and wheelchairs entered our world. It was at Disney World where I witnessed Gil, in his late thirties, finally allowing himself the carefree childhood denied to him by years of unsuccessful searching for love. There at Disney World I shared his newly rediscovered adolescent joy, both of us screaming through the darkness of Space Mountain, or nervously laughing before the elevator drop at the Tower of Terror.

Shortly following his death, it was a whim for me to purchase a brick in Gil's name on the Magic Kingdom Walk of Fame. He has an engraved marker skirting the path along the white sands overlooking the Disney's Grand Floridian Resort & Spa. This brick acknowledges the joy Gil found there. It is not a gravestone substitution; it simply states Gil's name and date of death, with a graphic of Mickey's white-gloved hands forming the shape of a heart. Gil's engraved name belongs in that uplifting kingdom of castles; and not in a solemn Zion of monuments, such as the cemetery in which I sat that day.

Loneliness slowly subsided. The sun had traveled a good distance along the cloudless, cornflower-blue sky, and I realized it was time for me to return to the writers' conference afternoon session. Where had the morning gone? Why had I not been writing? Or had I been composing through the mirror of my mind?

Hesitating, I surveyed the cemetery one last time as I righted my bicycle from its resting position. I slowly straddled it with a renewed feeling of peace. The warmth of the black padding on the handlebars felt reenergizing to my hands. A robin precariously perched on the stone obelisk designated "Milliken" captured my full attention. Ever since the morning of Gil's death, the robin carried the power to instantly remind me of Gil.

Gil, I can feel you.

I stared at the robin looking back at me with head cocked.

I can sense your presence, and I now know exactly where to find you.

"Gil?" My voice of revelation broke the wooded silence. Was the robin my omen? He reinforced the adage that "all things change, and all things remain the same." This bird was here with me each year, although migrating with the seasons. Gil would also be with me each year, even though he, too, migrated from my life.

Sitting firmly on the bicycle seat, I was now ready to continue my journey along the New Hampshire hills, and along the roads of life, with newly found contentment. I realized it was possible to continue a relationship with Gil throughout the remainder of my life, by keeping his memory always in my heart.

"NOTHING BUT HEARTACHES"

Hospice Volunteer Training
Session Eight:
Termination with Patient and Family

November 1, 1993

"Tonight's talk is a hard one. You've developed a relationship with a patient over time; possibly the two of you became very close. Sometimes that relationship carries over to the patient's family members. Tonight, I tell you your patient died."

No, Arlene. It's too soon. Gil can't die yet.

"Every situation is unique, but chances are you're now officially terminated with the case."

No, Arlene. It's not that easy. No one can just walk away.

"Of course, oftentimes you may attend the funeral for closure. And we also offer a weekly volunteer support group meeting so that you can talk about what's going on with your case, or how to handle the ending of a case."

No, Arlene. Our end is a long way away.

"Hospice maintains a professional relationship with the surviving family over the following year, and we're there for them in whatever capacity they choose to use us. So, we now need to talk about the volunteer's coping skills with saying goodbye."

No, Arlene. I'm not ready to say goodbye.

"Let me show you a short film about saying goodbye."

Florida

The Month of February 1996

His mother phoned one hot June day in 1994. She called not to schedule a visit with Gil, but to drop her latest bomb.

"Son, I'm flying to Florida next week to buy a mobile home." There was nonchalance in her tone.

She had answered a classified advertisement in the newspaper describing the mobile home.

His mother returned home to New England from the impulsive, three-day mobile-home-buying trip 1,000 miles south, now the owner of a trailer at a mobile home park and marina in Florida.

She called to tell Gil all about her trip. I did not understand his mother, or her gradual – but definite – distancing of herself from her son. Why couldn't she come for a visit and tell him this information in person?

"Why did you buy a trailer in Florida?" Gil asked in disbelief, but not total surprise. "Do you plan to move to Florida, use it for vacation, or rent it out?"

Her answer was always the same to Gil's repeatedly asked questions regarding the subject. "Son, it's an investment. And don't call it a trailer; it's a mobile *home.*" Her tone became defensive around the subject. "Property is a good thing to own, wherever."

His mother was a part of my life only because she was a part of Gil's. I did not like the way she moved through life. I accepted her. She was not the portrait of the martyred woman she attempted to draw for the world. She knew I gave Gil things that she could not, and that made his mother and me natural antagonists in life.

His mother continued her telephone conversation with Gil. "Son, are you boys planning to go to South Carolina and Disney World in January?" She waited for the answer she already knew. "Why don't you spend a few days at the mobile home with me to help set it up?" I could tell from Gil's look that she was asking for something of which I would not approve.

Without asking me, Gil mechanically answered, "Okay. We can do that."

Our plans for a relaxing vacation were altered by one maternal phone call. It was only June, but I began dreading the January trip to the trailer.

The photograph she brought back of the unadorned white metal box passing for a home had whetted Gil's curiosity regarding his mother's "investment."

His desire, before he died, was to see his mother happily settled for once in her life. Consequently, mother and son spent much energy that summer and fall on the phone, discussing her planned renovations. I wondered if this could be where his mother might finally find some grounding in her life.

January soon arrived. After two relaxing weeks of doing nothing on the beaches of South Carolina, we reloaded our luggage into Gil's Honda and drove to Florida. Gil had told his mother we would be there for only a few days, on our way to Orlando.

We easily located the mobile home park. The park was a grid of one-lane streets. Endless metal rectangles were positioned calculated distances apart. Each trailer was personalized with its own hideous motif. In comparison to the beer can creations and other lawn ornaments decorating the small lots, a plastic pink flamingo here and a manatee mailbox there were considered tasteful. The park's only redeeming features were the nearby creek and marina. Walking the weathered gangplanks and looking at the boats and the creek's wildlife relaxed Gil.

His mother was not due to arrive until the following morning. Tentatively, I unloaded our luggage from the car while Gil located the hidden key. As the flimsy metal door swung inward, our senses were assaulted: the emanating musty odor; the rust-colored, traffic-worn, stained shag carpet; and the confining, dingy, cream-colored, Formica-paneled walls, stained yellow from years of trapped cigarette smoke. The walls were still littered with the *tchotchkes* of someone else's life.

It was obvious Death had visited this trailer. The heir unloaded it on Gil's mother, without even bothering to clean it – neither emotionally nor hygienically. I asked Gil if he would be more comfortable staying at the Holiday Inn just a block away. He declined, mesmerized by the remains of the furnishings, all broken and mismatched – articles even

Goodwill might refuse for donation.

Over the past six months, Gil's mother had chosen to portray this trailer as an "investment." Her "future refuge" from Gil's disease and death was how I described her purchase. Gil needed to be embraced by the upbeat surroundings of life, not this crypt. However grim the surroundings were to us, this trailer had likely been a comfortable home for the previous occupant. If so, I hoped whoever it was had died peacefully here.

The kitchen and bathroom were filthy. The nesting mouse family was not happy to be displaced as we reactivated the corroding pink refrigerator. The furnace refused to ignite. I reminded myself we had only today to ourselves in this tomb before his mother's arrival, followed by two days of putting up with his mother in the cramped environment. We would then be free to escape to Disney World. *I can do it. I can do it. I can do it.* Those three words became my mantra.

Gil's immediate mission was to make the trailer as homey and welcoming as he could for his mother's arrival. We were off to Target for cleaning supplies, Circuit City for a vacuum and television, and Winn-Dixie for groceries. We had less than twenty-four hours to transform this trailer into a home – not so much comfort for our short duration, but hominess for his mother's potential long-range contentment.

We were scheduled to meet his mother at the airport the following morning. She probably could have walked to the mobile home park; I could almost see the control towers through the palm trees as I surveyed this foreign world from the tiny, oval trailer window. Gil and I shouted to each other over the deafening roar of the arriving and departing jets as we scrutinized our home-decorating efforts. Gil perfected last-minute touches one final time before her arrival.

Thoroughly exhausted by the end of the day, we opened the soiled, lumpy, plaid-patterned sofa bed. Our reward for our day's efforts was a bunched up, paper-thin, stained mattress. I closed my eyes, sucked in the air that reeked of cleaning products, and swore to myself I would never, ever return to this trailer.

We met his mother the following morning. After a brief embrace, she centered her conversation on the trailer. Not once did she inquire about our trip or Gil's health. I answered her ravings in a voice only I could hear.

"I can't believe I was talked into buying this mobile home." She started her litany of complaints.

I do not recall anyone forcing you to make the purchase.

"The seller never took me around the park to show me the other homes that were for sale."

Why would he? He was attempting to sell his trailer to you.

"He just took advantage of me and my money."

Same old story.

"I know I was overcharged."

As usual.

"This place is a dump."

You've got that right.

"Maybe I should sue him."

Why not?

"I should put this mobile home up for sale right now and buy a nicer one."

I cannot believe that you would ever say that aloud to me. So predictable.

For two days, that was all we heard from his mother, how she had been "had by life." I could not break it to Gil, but I did not think Florida was where his mother would be peacefully settled. I wondered if such a place existed at all.

For two mornings I drove his mother in Gil's car all over town so she could buy new furnishings, kitchen china, utensils, and glassware. For two afternoons, I suggested she rest from shopping so that I could escape with Gil for a little quiet time alone at a nearby beach. Those two afternoons alone with Gil became the only memory I cherished from our brief stay with his mother in Florida.

The time soon came for us to depart for Disney World, leaving his mother the rest of the week to fend for herself before returning to New Hampshire. She insisted we stay out the week with her so that she would not be alone and would be able to get around comfortably in our car; she had not rented a vehicle for herself during her stay. Kissing his mother goodbye, Gil declined, saying it would be the perfect opportunity for her to meet some of her neighbors, and she would discover how wonderful living on her own here could be. As expected, she resented being deserted.

Ten months later, on a frosty October morning, Gil's mother called him with the fallout news. She did not inquire as to her son's health status; she just blurted her update.

"Son, your brother and I have decided to sell everything and move to the mobile home the first of November." I saw Gil's puzzled look as he listened to his mother, although I did not yet know the reason.

"That's less than a month away. Why move now?" I heard him say the word "move." My suspicions had become reality.

"There's no sense having the mobile home unoccupied." She began to defend her reason for the sudden move. "Your brother can do the remodeling work."

He should do the remodeling work. He had been living with their mother since Gil's AIDS diagnosis, suddenly appearing out of nowhere. His reappearance into their family instantly shifted her attention from her sick son to her well son. Gil's brother was a few years older than Gil. His mother supported her live-in son, treating this man in his late forties as though he were still her adolescent.

"But why now? Right before the holidays?" Gil continued to express his disbelief.

"Son, we need to leave before the snow comes. Don't worry." Her sentence pace quickened as she attempted to calm Gil's questioning. "You'll be down to see us after the holidays. You boys can stay with us for a whole month." The cordless phone allowed Gil to pace the carpet in the center of the living room until he had had enough.

"I'll call you later."

The trailer had been uninhabited for the year and one-half since her purchase. For the previous four years, his mother and brother had denied Gil's disease. Recently, they could not even fulfill a commitment to drive an hour to visit with Gil once a week. By moving to Florida, distancing themselves even more, they would no longer need to make their weekly excuses for not coming. I believed they saw Gil's rapidly approaching death and could no longer deal with his dying. At the time, I did not fully grasp the way people might handle the death and dying of others.

They sold all their apartment furnishings within two weeks. They packed and shipped the few remaining mementos, framed pictures, kitchenware, and linens. All that was left to do was to load to capacity their ancient Oldsmobile with a television, clothing, and luggage. On the first of November, his mother and brother headed south. Were they coping with Gil's impending death in their own way? They never saw the pain of their departure in Gil's eyes. They were taking care of themselves, and I was left to take care of Gil, alone, for his five remaining months.

Throughout November and December, they called from Florida. The distant conversations were full of weather reports and current temperatures, what improvements his brother had done to the trailer, and how much they looked forward to our upcoming visit in January. They never inquired about Gil's condition; the conversations always centered on their new life in Florida.

Our month-long visit south approached. We would fly this year because Gil could no longer tolerate the long drive. The planned itinerary began in Florida with a few days at the trailer with his mother and brother. From there, we would rent a car and head to South Carolina for the month. At the end of our vacation, we would return to Florida for a few days, for one last visit with his family, and then fly home to

New Hampshire.

However, the plans changed when we arrived in Florida. Gil's condition was rapidly declining. Once the plane landed, he was too fatigued to travel elsewhere. I was now destined to spend our entire month-long "vacation" in the trailer with his mother and brother; the sty, one year before, I had vowed never to visit again.

Each morning, I rode a rusty, second-hand exercise bicycle stationed on the concrete driveway in an attempt to maintain some sanity. Inside, his mother was spending one-on-one time with Gil, at my request. Pedaling furiously, I reviewed the daily routine that had already emerged in the few days we had been there.

During breakfast, his mother would compile a list of items she "urgently" needed to purchase that day. She and his brother would soon be out the door, shopping for the entire morning. They would return in time for his mother to prepare lunch. Following our meal, I would ask to borrow their Oldsmobile to take Gil for a ride, anywhere for a change of scenery for him and an escape for me. His mother then prepared dinner. Following the meal, the family settled in for an entire evening of television, starting every night with *COPS* and ending with the eleven o'clock news.

This daily schedule never varied, and it was driving me insane. My heart rate increased as I furiously pedaled the bicycle each morning, thinking of our precious time together wasting away.

Thankfully, everyone respected my request not to be disturbed during my one hour on the bicycle each morning. Only Gil was allowed to break that rule. On the third morning, he tentatively approached me. His short-sleeve shirt had a pattern of brightly colored tropical birds, his shorts a clashing lime green. On his feet were turquoise espadrilles, and on his face a look of solemn concern.

"What are you going to say to my mother when she asks us to stay longer?" He blurted this to me with no prelude.

"What do you mean, Gil? Why would she ask?"

I was surprised she had waited three days before making the anticipated request.

"Oh, you know how she is."

Sadly, I did know.

"And you know what my answer will be."

I needed to be firm, and Gil needed to hear that tone in my voice. He meandered toward the trailer.

From the bicycle, I surveyed the garden I was in the process of planting on their barren trailer lot. I had named it "Gil's Garden." It was my contribution to add some beauty to their life so that maybe they might establish some roots here in Florida, as Gil had hoped. Mainly, the garden gave me something to do during the hours of being trapped there. In this temperate zone, I was beginning to familiarize myself with Florida plants that I could add to the freshly dug garden beds: Queen Sago palm, *podocarpus, croton,* Chinese holly, hibiscus, oleander, and *ixora* – plants I could not cultivate in our New Hampshire gardens. I was sure Gil's family did not appreciate my efforts, but I wanted to believe they did.

I was planting the hedge of oleanders, after my cycle workout, when his mother approached. Her request was blunt. "Andrew, do you have a hundred dollars, so I can buy wallpaper for the kitchen?"

One hundred dollars for wallpaper? Neither of them was working. His mother had been briefly employed at a nursing home shortly after the move to Florida. His bother's "occupation" was remodeling the trailer.

"I'm sorry. You know our situation." I attempted politeness. "I only budgeted enough money to spend on food during our stay. Would you rather I spent a week's worth of grocery money on wallpaper?" I knew what her answer would be to that question. Her life priorities were skewed. She would pick the wallpaper.

She had, once again, overstepped her boundary with me.

That afternoon, Gil and I forfeited our usual peaceful afternoon ride for a wallpaper-shopping trip with his mother. She frantically searched the rolls, but she could find nothing that suited her. I was relieved. She suggested another store. Gil told her he was just too tired to continue. We returned home empty-handed.

I still needed an afternoon getaway for sanity. I asked if I might borrow the Oldsmobile to visit a nearby state park. Gil usually would want to join me, but he was too drained from the day of shopping. It might be important for mother and son to spend some time alone, without me. I would be away from the trailer, and his brother would be out for the afternoon. Maybe, if the two of them were completely alone, she might tell Gil the words he ached to hear from his mother. He wanted to hear her say that she was happy and feeling settled and that his illness was much more life-threatening than any illness she professed to be suffering. He longed to hear her sincerely say, "I love you." I left the two of them for the afternoon, hoping those words would come from her heart.

I will never know what transpired that afternoon while I trekked the paths of the reserve. When I returned, his brother sat dazed in front of the television, while his mother was giving Gil a back rub. It was a rare act of caring that I seldom had seen her perform since our arrival. Perhaps it had been good for me to allow them a private afternoon.

I noticed it was slightly past the time to give Gil his medications, one of four daily dosings.

"Gil, time for your pills." I gently intruded upon son and mother.

"Tell Andrew I gave them to you already." Her snapping-turtle persona suddenly reemerged.

There was no response from Gil; he seemed to be enjoying his mother's touch on his body. I quietly retreated to the dining room to check his pillbox. I had come with an itemized schedule of the multitude of his daily medications. The day we arrived, I had sat with his mother at the dining room table and explained to her my system of dispensing the medications into the pill box organizer that stored his medications for a week at a time. I also made her aware that the medications must be secreted from Gil so that he did not mistakenly overdose on any of his medications, as he had done on our trip to Nantucket. She showed no interest in the system I had perfected. For years I had attempted to include her as a part of her son's medical care; she rarely seemed to want to participate. She disputed every medical decision Gil made, holding me responsible for his choices.

I double-checked the pillbox to determine whether his mother might have given Gil the medications from a wrong compartment. The scheduled pills had not been removed from their compartment.

"Gil's pills are still in the organizer." I spoke gently as I reentered the room. "Did you take the pills from the bottles instead?" I tried my best to ask without accusation.

"I told you I gave Gil his meds." Resembling a tortoise, her head would extend, snap out the words, and then retract.

"I'm only confirming the dosages." I attempted to keep my voice calm for Gil's benefit.

"You don't believe me?" Snap, snap.

"Did your mother give you medication recently?" I reeled from her tone and redirected my question to Gil.

"Andrew, I don't think so," he answered. I knew Gil did not want to be a part of this.

"I'm asking you one more time." I attempted to reason with her as I again redirected my line of questioning. "Did you, or did you not, give Gil his medications?"

"You don't believe me when I told you that I did?" Snap, snap, snap.

"I wish I could have that trust in you." *But I certainly do not.*

It was time for a referee, however impartial he might not be. His brother was hanging in the doorway, eager to escape the confrontation that was going on.

"I need to have you ask your mother whether she gave Gil his medications." My serious tone appeared to touch a part of him I had not yet discovered.

"Andrew needs to know if you gave Gil his medications." His no-nonsense tone matched mine.

Mother glared at son, rather than at me, as the words spewed from her lips.

"I refuse to give Gil any of those pills. It's the medications that are killing him." Snap, snap, snap, snap. "I've been telling him all these years that the only thing he should be taking is B-12 injections because he's merely anemic." Snap, snap, snap, snap, snap. "No. I did not give Gil the pills that Andrew makes him take." Snap. Neck retracted, she marched out of the room.

"You're a nurse," I called after her. "Gil is taking large doses of morphine four times daily. I think you know, as a nurse, what would happen to Gil if you suddenly withdrew his scheduled morphine." She just kept walking, out the door of the trailer, not wanting to hear anything I had to say.

She may have felt newly found power over us. We were in her territory now, not in the comfort of our home. For the remainder of the night, she refused to say one word to me. Florida's balmy winds suddenly became unseasonably chilled. It was time for us to leave.

During our regular evening walk around the maze of garish mobile homes, made even more so by the moonlight reflecting their pleated metal sides, I suggested to Gil that we cut our trip short and head home. I impressed upon him the need to be near his medical support system and to be closer to our circle of friends. He refused. He would not leave until his mother simply told him the words he needed to hear.

The following morning, four of us sat around the gray-speckled Formica and stainless-steel kitchen table as we ate a silent breakfast. Mother and brother could not leave the table soon enough for their morning of errands. His mother had spent the entire time at the table compiling her list. Alone with Gil, I pleaded my case once again of how important it was for us to go home. He once again dismissed my concerns, and he asked if we could visit a nearby botanical garden that afternoon, after his mother and brother returned with the car.

Upon our entering the tropical garden, Gil immediately pointed to the row of wheelchairs lined against the wall. "Andrew, would you mind pushing me in one of those today?" I was surprised by his request. "I want to see how it feels to ride in one." It had been only a year since our last visit here. The change in Gil's health over that one year was clearly obvious to me, as I assisted an "elderly" Gil into the wheelchair. There was also a noticeable redirection in Gil's spirits, most likely as a result of the previous day's confrontation between his mother and me.

When we returned to the trailer, his mother was sitting out front on a second-hand, mustard-colored, vinyl-upholstered restaurant chair that passed for lawn furniture. She was somewhat shielded from the street by my newly planted hedge of oleanders. She met our approach with, "I think it's time for you boys to go home."

These were not the words Gil needed to hear from his mother. His body reacted with a slumping of shoulders and that same pained look in his eyes I had witnessed when she had informed him of their sudden intention to move south, just months before. "Okay, Mother. Will tomorrow be soon enough?"

We were in the back seat of the Oldsmobile for one last ride. His mother and brother drove us to the airport. I could not help thinking, as we said our goodbyes, that it must be so hard for any mother to witness the progressing stages of death in her son. However, it seemed much more painful to share the agony of a son whose mother apparently refused to admit and participate in his dying.

That was the last time Gil saw his mother and brother – at the airport in Florida.

Letting Go of Gil's Baggage

March / April 1996

>*Dear Mom,*
>
>*I love you.*
>
>*Be good.*
>
>*Don't cause too much trouble.*
>
>*Don't lie too much.*
>
>*Try and get settled.*
>
>*Go on with your life.*
>
>*Remember I'm in a better place,*
>
>*And don't feel sorry for me.*

Gil dictated to me these eight lines, simply stated, in a letter to his mother a week before the coma, when he was too weak, or too disinterested, to write.

Four days after Gil's death, I, too, needed to write to Gil's family, a thousand miles away. I had had enough of their disturbing telephone calls following Gil's death. There were things I needed to make clear to them.

Within minutes of Gil's death, I made my first phone call – it was to his family. What I expected to be a very difficult conversation, informing a mother of her son's death, became merely a brief exchange of information. She claimed to be too upset to talk at the moment. I could understand; I, too, was distraught. I told her I would check in again later. That evening, I called to see how they both were doing. I wanted to share my grief with them. Again, they were unavailable to talk.

The next afternoon, only one day after Gil's death, his brother called me.

"Andrew, you need to take care of yourself." He spoke with such authority.

"I know. I'm trying." I had not yet begun to think of myself.

"You've been through a lot, and you still have much to take care of." What did he know of what I had been through? What was he saying I needed to take care of?

"I know." Or thought I knew. "I have some things Gil set aside for both of you. I'll send them later this week, along with Gil's ashes. He wanted his mother to have these things."

"Don't send Gil's ashes or anything to us here." He now spoke with the edge of warning. "We'll be coming back to New Hampshire soon."

"I hope your mother is doing okay. Bye." I slammed the phone down in disbelief.

Not one word of comfort from his family. I craved such words from both of them. Not one question from them regarding the execution of Gil's wishes: cremation plans, scattering of Gil's remains, memorial, or chosen destination for memorial contributions. These were topics they had brushed aside whenever brought up for discussion. Their reply was always the same: "You know Gil's wishes."

Not one offer from his family to assist with Gil's final arrangements. Rather, I began receiving their businesslike calls, the calls Gil had warned me would come from them someday.

His brother called again the following afternoon.

"Andrew, just calling to see how the life insurance paperwork is going."

"What paperwork?" I knew exactly what he meant. "I haven't made those calls yet." I had not even received Gil's remains.

I knew exactly where these daily conversations were leading.

To avoid any more conversations with Gil's brother, I let the answering machine handle all their calls. On the fourth afternoon, I realized it was time for an unlisted number. I needed to put an end to these communications from Florida.

I had just inherited what Gil described as his "baggage." I remembered Gil saying to me on our first date, "Most people come with baggage in their lives, but I have to let you know up front. I've got garbage." He recognized it and could admit it. I could now acknowledge it, too.

I realized I could now leave Gil's baggage at the station and take the train to my next destination without it. Gil would say, "I wish I could stuff all this family garbage of mine in a trash bag, heave it into the dumpster, and let it be taken away forever." I did just that for both of us in the two letters sent to Florida – Gil's dictated letter and mine.

Gil had put together a small collection of family mementos that he personally chose, just weeks before his death, to have returned to his mother and brother after he died. The items were of no monetary value: some family photographs; a carving set that his biological father, a chef, had owned; a two-dollar bill; an inexpensive print of a leaping cat his brother had given Gil one birthday not long before; and the then-empty, small, corked pottery container. Gil had requested I place some of his cremated remains in this crock to send to his mother.

I had prepared all these items for UPS shipping, except for three: the pottery container; Gil's eight-line letter addressed to his mother, to which I added the explanation: "Gil dictated this letter prior to his death and made me promise to send it to you." There was also a letter, addressed to his mother and brother, which I had drafted angrily in the days following Gil's death.

My eight-page letter to them was more detailed than Gil's eight lines of dying wisdom to his mother. My letter itemized every hurtful incident that had transpired over the past eight years. Eight pages of injustices: their abandonment of shared caregiving duties; his mother's continual questioning of Gil's medical choices and the credentials of his physician; their sudden move from New Hampshire to Florida just months before his death; and their intent to return immediately following his death. Also listed was the inability of his mother, right up to the end of his life, to give Gil the unconditional love that he sought from her; and, ultimately, the validation from his mother that his disease was much more painful and life-ending than any items on the menu of illnesses she professed to have, ranging from diabetes to high blood pressure.

Rereading my letter, I realized I could not send it to them, as accurate as it was. They would categorically deny every point I raised. My letter would anger and rally them all the more. But I needed to send my letter; they needed to know the anger and disappointment I was feeling toward them both. The telephone interrupted my dilemma. It was the funeral home informing me that I might come for Gil's remains. That afternoon, I brought home Gil's ashes.

I rose early the next morning to perform a ritual. I hastily collected the necessary items: my letter; a Pyrex baking pan; a silver serving spoon; and the burgundy velvet sack, tied with a drawstring, containing the blue cardboard box sheltering Gil's remains. Supervised by the rising sun, I took this collection of items outside. That morning was the first time I viewed, and touched, Gil's remains. I slowly scooped them, spoonful by spoonful, from the twist-tied plastic bag within the cardboard box into the gray and blue, salt-glazed pottery container. This was the receptacle Gil had chosen, with his mother, more than a year earlier, expressly for this purpose. I filled his makeshift urn, leaving a header space of one inch.

I took my letter and reread aloud all eight pages one last time. I spat out the words; they froze before me, suspended in the vapor of the chilled April morning air. Holding the letter over the Pyrex pan, I struck a match that provided a little pocket of warmth around my trembling hands. The flame touched the lower, right-hand corner of my letter. I watched the pages curl and blacken. They fell into the clear baking dish, bits of words still readable, ghostly white against blackened paper; words describing disappointment and disbelief.

I stirred the remains of the letter with my forefinger and let them loose into the cold breeze. Then I poured some of those letter ashes into the container of Gil's ashes. The urn was now full. Corking the pottery container tightly, I gently, and lovingly, rolled the remains of Gil between my palms for what seemed a very long time. This ritual was my way of sending his family my letter, releasing it forever from my world.

Into the box of his family memorabilia, I placed the pottery jar. Affixed to it was a copy of Gil's obituary from the newspaper, along with his eight dictated lines to his mother. Clear package tape sealed the Florida-bound corrugated-cardboard box, and it was mailed that afternoon.

When I got home, I wrote his family a new letter; this one his family would soon receive separately by mail:

The time has come for us to say goodbye.

Goodbye to Gil and goodbye to each other. Saying goodbye is hard, but it is also necessary. Saying goodbye to Gil has been the hardest thing for me to do in my entire life.

We must all heal from Gil's passing in whatever way it takes. I hope you will understand that in order for me to move on in my life, I am saying goodbye to you both; and in order for me to do that, I want to let you know clearly what that means.

To move on and heal from Gil's passing, I am asking that you respect my wish for you to discontinue any future telephone calls or visits to my home.

Should you need to contact me for any reason, a message may be left with my attorney.

Goodbye,
Andrew

This letter finally allowed me to let go of Gil's baggage. The garbage he warned me he would bring along with him.

———◦◦◦———

See Appendix J:
End-of-Life Coaching Exercise...
RECONCILIATION, page 252.

"THE HAPPENING"

Hospice Volunteer Training
Session Nine:
Graduation

November 8, 1993

Graduation night: Diplomas. Hugs. Congratulations. We had all successfully completed the hospice training. We were official Seacoast Hospice volunteers. Food for our final evening together was pot luck, and Gil had insisted on sending me with his marinated chicken wings. I never understood, never asked, and will never be able to tell anyone what ingredients made them that unnatural reddish color. They were always the hit at any gathering, and tonight was no exception. Gil felt a part of the celebration by sending me with his wings. He deserved to be represented after vicariously experiencing the nine training weeks with me. We were both graduating to a higher level of understanding the dying process.

"Attention, everyone," Arlene announced. "While you're grazing over food, I need to pull each one of you aside individually for your exit interview."

"So, Andrew. How did you hold up for the nine weeks?" Arlene asked me with concern.

"It was more than I could have asked for. Much more than either Gil or I could have expected."

"We're going to make another exception for you, Andrew. No payback volunteer hours until the timing is right."

"What do you mean by 'timing?'"

"Your life is full right now. Take the entire lessons home with you. Make Gil your twenty-four-hour-a-day hospice patient."

"No, Arlene. I need to do something in return for hospice now. I don't want to be treated as an exception."

"Take some time. We'll meet again in a month or two, sometime down the road." I flashed back nine weeks to her "hospice policies and procedures."

"No. I've got to do something now. Bereavement."

"What are you offering, Andrew?"

"I want to write bereavement letters, at home, not taking away any precious time with Gil. I'll do them while he watches television, while he naps, when he gets sick, after he dies." I started to cry.

"Andrew, I say let's do it. But strictly on a trial basis. You can stop anytime you need to. Come to my office tomorrow morning. We'll get you started. You know, it's been difficult keeping up with the letters lately. You're probably just what we need."

I came home relieved. Training was finished. I daydreamed of rescuing their bereavement letter program, improving it, adding new touches... and before I knew it, Gil was home from work.

"Are congratulations in order?"

"Yes, but aren't you going to ask me what we talked about tonight?" I missed his usual greeting that I had come to expect over the past eight weeks.

"Why ask? I know that everyone was requesting my recipe for the chicken wings all night. And you don't even know one ingredient that goes into them. Do you?"

"I can name the most important one: love."

See Appendix K:
End-of-Life Coaching Exercise...
BECOME A DEATH AND DYING ADVOCATE, page 253.

"REFLECTIONS"

Epilogue:
"No New..."

April 1996

With the bathroom mirror before me, I declared to my now gaunt reflection, "No new cars, no new relationships, no new homes." And I meant it. I'd been through too much. I planned to give myself at least a year of "no more loss" in my life.

I surprised myself with the force of this declaration, spoken aloud, as I pumped the remaining essence of the Calvin Klein "Eternity for Men" cologne onto my chest, noticing gray chest hairs that seemed to have appeared overnight. Tilting in all directions the once-filled bottle of amber liquid, I wanted to inhale every last ambrosial drop, one last time.

"Eternity." It was Gil's fragrance. Now it was empty. Gone. As was Gil. Just days before. I filled my lungs deeply with as much of the aroma as I could. Nothing is eternal.

Tears blurred my morning reflection in the bathroom mirror. Vignettes of our years as "GILANDANDREW" flashed in no ordered sequence before my mind's eye.

It had been twelve short months since making that morning declaration. Did I feel I did not deserve change during my self-imposed year of grieving and healing? How did I feel today, knowing I broke all three of my rules, one by one? Was it permissible to break these vows within the first twelve months? I stared at my clear reflection in the bathroom mirror, thinking over the changes made during the past year. I had a newly purchased bottle of "Eternity" in my hand. It had been a year since a bottle of his scent had resided in the house.

NO NEW CARS

I clearly remembered the conversation I had with Gil not long before he died. He would start the exchange, as if the topic had some immediacy. Yet, I knew it was more out of his concern about my survival after he was gone.

"We need to get a larger, safer car." He claimed it was difficult for him to get in and out of his little Honda. Also, if he should ever need a wheelchair? It would never fit.

"Gil, we cannot afford a new car." He was collecting disability and social security income; I was working part time. I attempted to justify reasons for not buying a new car.

Yet, how Gil had salivated over our neighbor's recently acquired second-hand Volvo station wagon. "Three years old." "Only 30,000 miles." "In mint condition." These three phrases began to sound like a daily mantra from Gil's lips. Was the practical, purse-string-holding, Yankee side of me denying Gil the comfort of a larger vehicle? Was I refusing him the peace of mind that together we could find a larger, safer car that would take care of me after he was gone? Was that the real issue? If we were to purchase a new car together, would it prevent my potential guilty feelings when I eventually purchased a new car, at some future date after his death?

Ironically, only months after Gil's death, our Volvo neighbors needed to sell their car. They had been offered an overseas job transfer.

That evening I had one of those one-sided conversations with Gil. Wherever he might be.

Gil, I know you've been gone for only four months, but is it too soon to think about getting a new car?

There was silence in the living room as I paced the vacant spot where those ghostly indentations remained in the Oriental rug, telltale marks, where his hospital bed once commanded attention.

We should've done it while you were alive.

There was silence in the dining room as I placed the Fiesta dishes on the round table, still setting it for two.

Can you give me a sign that it's the right thing to do?

None. There was silence in our queen-sized, four-poster bed as I fell asleep on what was always "my side of the bed."

I awoke the following morning to a rainstorm.

The storm eventually abated and, in combination with the sun, presented me with a full arc rainbow doming the backyard. A rainbow. Gil's beloved ribbons of prisms. Was this the sign from Gil giving me his permission to buy the Volvo?

I thought yes, each time I was seated at the wheel.

NO NEW RELATIONSHIPS

I remembered a conversation with Gil that occurred just after he had been diagnosed with HIV, years prior to his death.

"Come to the pharmacy with me today." He wanted me to meet his pharmacist, who he thought was gorgeous and might be gay. "The two of you would be perfect together."

"Gil, how could you think such a thing?" Why would he think such a thing?

"Andrew, I want you to be loved, and happy, after I'm gone." He spoke with sincerity.

"I'll be fine." End of discussion.

So how could I consider any relationships, just months after Gil's passing? Five months after his death, I was having a monologue with Gil.

Gil, it's too soon to open my heart to anyone else.

There was silence from the patio deck as I mounted my bicycle, surveying the palette of flowers we had planted together.

Am I supposed to say to this person, "My year of mourning hasn't yet expired. Come back in a few months?"

There was silence, except for the whooshing air, as I punishingly pedaled my bicycle to near-exhaustion.

I know you'd approve, Gil. He's not your pharmacist, but a rabbi.

There was silence from the garage as I hung my bicycle on the red utility hooks.

I had pictured a rabbi as an old man dressed in black, with long curls and an unkempt, scraggly beard, wearing a prayer shawl and a *yarmulke* – an image from my teenage experiences of celebrating classmates' *Bar Mitzvahs.*

However, Rabbi Lev Baesh did not fit my preconceived image. I knew this man not as a rabbi, but as "The Frequent Purchaser of Fruit Trees." He was a customer at the garden center, where I had been work-ing part time during Gil's illness and then full time after Gil's death. Throughout the spring following Gil's death, this man had repeatedly purchased many varieties of fruit trees: apples, nectarines, peaches, pears, plums, and cherries – sweet and sour. Had I ever speculated on this man's sexual preference? Perhaps. Did I ever acknowledge this man's religion? It was obvious by the *yarmulke.* However, I had never enter-tained the thought that this man, buying too many fruit trees, could be my potential life partner, my new soulmate. It was too soon after Gil's death for me to even think such things. Fortunately, Rabbi Lev had taken the responsibility of considering the possibility.

On one of his visits to the garden center, I initiated a conversation on topics other than horticultural. We spoke briefly amid the remain-ing rows of potted fruit trees. Our relationship started, as the conversa-tion ended, with his sighing, "I'm glad we finally connected. I'm running out of room for planting any more fruit trees."

———◦◦◦———

NO NEW HOMES

I thought back to our discussion of what would become of our home once Gil was no longer here. We had discussed what life might be like for me after he was gone.

"Gil, I would never sell our house." I assured him that if I should move for any reason, I would rent it.

"Don't sell unless it's for 'big bucks,'" he would advise me whenever we had this conversation.

I found myself looking over a lease agreement eleven months after Gil departed the home we had shared.

And I still conversed with Gil, months after his departure.

Gil, a realtor is searching for an available condo to rent for her clients. I was not actively looking to rent our home, but the opportunity presented itself.

There was silence from the living room as I scanned the collected treasures of our life together.

I've many memories here. I did. I do. But here, also, were the painful reminders of your last month here.

There was silence as I kneeled and scrubbed, once again, the stubborn, medication-colored urine stain on the carpet. It also marked where his hospital bed was once placed.

Someone is willing to pay "big bucks" for rent. Do you approve, Gil?

There was silence as I scanned the memorabilia placed on the piano, still remaining on display.

I broke the room's silence with my phone call to the potential renters. "I have the rental agreement ready for your signature."

———◦◦◦———

Was it a valid concept that major, life-altering decisions should not be made so soon after the death of your life partner? I attempted to give myself one full year to delay such weighty decisions. But can my grief be measured by a self-imposed, predetermined time interval? Would one year be long enough? Or, would one year be too long? Did I believe that exactly one year, to the date, after Gil's passing I miraculously would be healed and ready to move on with my life?

Grief is an ongoing process that will always be with me. Grief should lessen with time. Did I feel guilt, or regret, for making any of these transitions? I supposed I could allow myself to feel unfaithful to Gil, but I did not. The truth was I had been grieving for more than five years.

Grief did not start the moment Gil died. It began the day of Gil's HIV diagnosis, with the realization that our life together, and shared dreams of a future, would wilt and die. Grief was not a new emotion for me, commencing on the morning of March 30, 1996.

I continued to have my daily conversations with Gil. I talked of our past, the present, and my future.

In retrospect, Gil taught me that death is the ultimate teacher. He made me see how precious, and brief, life is. Not to waste a single moment. Not to "sweat the small things." Not to close myself off to life's continued offerings.

However, I walked a difficult five-year journey. I have grown, and I have changed from my experience. I will never be the same person that I was.

I am thankful to have been blessed with Gil's final gift: allowing me to share our stories.

———⊙⊙⊙———

There was no longer silence in the bathroom as I conversed with Gil, generously dousing myself with the essence of the newly purchased, full bottle of "Eternity." Gil lives on, through my writing, through these memoirs that, until now, had been reflected only through the mirror of my mind.

The Memory Book

The memory book has become a wonderful storybook, with contributions from seventy-one authors. I have browsed through it many times during the year following Gil's death. On the one-year anniversary of his journey, I read it cover-to-cover for the first time. Reading the memory book, either in its entirety or as stand-alone personal essays, has become my continued connection to Gil, reflected through the eyes of others. I remember how this book came to be.

Jean was bringing lunch. I was apprehensive concerning her visit. A week before, we had scheduled this time together, just for the three of us. However, life could change drastically in just one week. I called early in the morning to let her know Gil was in a coma. I asked if she still would come for lunch. Her answer: "Of course."

Jean and I sat at the round, glass-topped dining room table.

Ironically, this small oak table painted Charleston Green, with two folding leaves, had been a topic of debate during my entire relationship with Gil. Two tables were involved in these discussions. My round table fit nicely in our small dining area but would seat only the two of us comfortably. Gil's larger, rectangular harvest table with two folding leaves would accommodate any larger number of guests. Our discussion for years was whether to find a replacement table with many removable leaves, which would allow one table to grow from small to large as needed. For special occasion meals over the years, I had done the table exchange, carting tables up and down the flight of stairs. Once assisted by Gil, and recently single-handedly, I would exchange my smaller, round table for his larger, rectangular table stored in the basement.

Gil's harvest table would comfortably seat eight. Not that my family, meshed with Gil's, was my idea of a cozy gathering. But this group became our collective family of origin, gathered around the harvest table for holidays, birthdays, and anniversaries. For eight years, Gil proposed we find a new dining room table. But a new table never became my priority, as I continued to do the table exchange, up and down the stairs, dozens of times each year, for eight years. It had become a familiar ritual. That day, as I prepared the small, round table for lunch with Jean, a larger table was the furthest thing from my mind; and it was now a moot subject between Gil and me.

Gil lay motionless on the hospital bed, just feet away from Jean and me. We sat at the round dining room table, its glass top reflecting the inside of my grandmother's Tiffany lamp hanging above. Our looks of wonder, concern, anxiety, caring, and love were reflected on that table-top. It must have been difficult for Jean to sit at that dining room table, as we talked and lunched. I had become comfortable with Gil's unmoving presence in the room. I could tell when our visitors were making the adjustment from Gil's usual verbal presence to merely his physical existence in the room. Jean attempted this transition by speaking of their past. Her history with Gil predated my time with him. Jean and I reminisced about lost days until our conversation eventually turned from the light to the heavy realities of that day.

I described to Jean my concept for creating a "memory book," a collection of personal writings from our friends that could be compiled into one special book. She was a graphic designer and immediately embraced my idea, offering her suggestions. Eventually, I felt comfortable enough in her presence to break down.

"Jean, some days I feel so overwhelmed." I had concerns about wanting to do the right things, carrying out Gil's wishes. "I can't consult with him anymore." I was feeling out of control with the situation.

She stroked my hand and reassured me that, even though Gil could no longer speak, he could hear our entire conversation and approved.

Our meal ended. It was time for Jean to return to work. It was time for me to return to my job of taking care of Gil. All thoughts of the memory book vanished with Jean's departure. There would be time to plan it later; today I had to be totally present for Gil.

That night, I dined alone at the round table, but I kept my eyes fixed on Gil. The phone interrupted the stillness of the room.

"Andrew, it's Jean." Her voice comforted me in my loneliness. "I couldn't get that memory book out of my head."

I tried to tell her that there was no need to rush it.

"Don't give it another thought. It's done." She told me she would bring it over soon, sometime in the next few days.

How brave of Jean to take on such a project I considered very personal. Could she design something from our brief conversation that would be acceptable to me? Wouldn't we need to discuss it in more detail? She knew what we liked, and I trusted her work.

A few days later, Jean gave me her prototype of the memory book. It measured 12 by 9 inches. The front and back covers consisted of heavy, brown, vertically corrugated paper. On the left-hand side, a pair of cocoa rawhide lacings bound the covers together. The lacings, tied in two large bows, were ample enough to accommodate the large collection of yet-to-be-contributed memory pages.

The paper for personal writings was the standard 8 ½ by 11 inches, off-white and subtlety flecked with muted browns and blues. There were eighteen horizontal lines provided for reflective writing. The page was adorned with three gray-shaded icons: the lower left hand corner, a radiating, smiling sun; off-center toward the right margin, a crescent moon; in the upper left corner, dominated by a large heart, pulsed the words "Memories of Gil." I loved what Jean had created. I presented the book to Gil, hoping he could see it, searching his face for a sign of approval. There was none.

———

I randomly thumbed through this collection of memory pages. Just holding the book reminded me of its evolution. The pages that came by mail, the pages brought to the celebration, and the straggler pages that continued to arrive during the ensuing year. Each of the bound seventy-one pages was a "personal snapshot" of Gil's life and spirit.

One memory page had no writings, but contained two photographs. Both were taken before my time with Gil. One pictured Gil dressed for a Halloween party as his idol, Diana Ross. He was outfitted in a black wig, huge hoop earrings, a rose-colored sleeveless dress, and black elbow-length gloves. He was seemingly unaware of the camera, with the frozen image of his arms, rhythmically flailing to the Motown Sound. The companion photo was of Gil and Dawn, who submitted these two visual memories. Both were sitting on a red-, white-, and blue-striped towel, stretched on the clean sands of Ogunquit Beach, Maine. The camera caught them in the process of removing their street shorts to reveal bikini bathing suits. Gil's bronzed skin played against his canary-yellow tank top and aqua-with-green, vertically striped Speedo suit. He looked happy and healthy in that photo: the image of the carefree Gil as he was when I first met him.

The next snapshot I encountered was more recent. It was of a trio: me, flanked by Gil on one side and our neighbor, Kaitlin, on the other. The guys were sporting winter beards, but Gil's facial hair did not mask the drawn look that was beginning to become more notice-able. Connie, who had introduced me to the concept of *Shiva* and the photographer of this memory moment, wrote, "I believe Gil was one of the sweetest, kindest men that I have known, and what a cook! This attached picture was taken at my house. We had a pot luck dinner; to me it represents a very happy time."

On another page a Polaroid photo was hidden by an attached large, red AIDS awareness ribbon. On the ribbon was written "Gil Ornelas 3-30-96," and a common pin kept the ribbon in its intended shape. "December 1993" was written on the bottom of the photo. This image was of Gil and me on our friend Patricia's couch; I was holding Gil very protectively in my arms. Again, we were both bearded during a differ-ent winter. Gil would keep a closely cut beard so that he would not need to shave. The developing, and spreading, molluscum virus that caused him much anguish made it difficult for him to shave over the raised patches of skin on his face. Gil looked gaunt in this photo taken three years before his death. He was wearing clashing reds – a short-sleeve T-shirt and sweatpants with "Ogunquit" trailing down one entire pant leg. Comfort ruled over fashion in his selection of clothes. Patricia had written, "My 'season' knowing Gil was much too short, but my memories of him will last my lifetime. Gourmet meals. Very few people have ever called me 'Patty,' but Gilly almost always did. I never told him, but I wish I had, how it always made me feel warm inside and loved."

Gil's cousin from his childhood past, with whom Gil had recently reconnected, attached a photograph taken decades before my time with Gil. It presented a childhood Gil, as she had known him. The faded image in rose tones, approaching sepia, depicted clashing floral patterns of the drapes, carpet, and couch. Two candy-filled, woven baskets and a spindly, potted Easter lily were arranged on a coffee table. Standing at attention with a big smile, dressed in a child's suit and tie, was the innocently smiling Gil. He was probably six years old. How Gil loved all holidays, and how Gil hated wearing a tie. She writes on her page, as if she could still address Gil directly, as if he were still alive and would read her written thoughts, "I remember you coming to your father's funeral. We talked about how strange our family was. You were treated like an outsider. I remember our sharing about our lives and why we were who we were." Her page revealed much from Gil's painful childhood.

A small clipped photo of a sunrise, through the silhouette of palm fronds, graced another page. There was not one person in this photo, submitted by our friend, Katrina. The strong solar symbol conjured a memory of a wonderful vacation to Hilton Head Island, South Carolina, with her and a group of friends. Katrina, who witnessed with me the intense intimacy of the moment of Gil's death, wrote, "Gil was and is such a gift to me. He had great wisdom and he lived it simply. One of our most profound talks was about simplifying my life, as he had, about coming home, spending time and energy with those you love, doing what you love, and putting those you love first in decisions to be made. Gil shared his secret to happiness with me."

Another photo captured Gil in a contemplative mood sitting in the uncomfortable, ornately sculpted Victorian chair in our living room. He was dressed in an off-white turtleneck, unbuttoned chamois-colored vest, beige slacks and socks, and gray Birkenstocks. My parents preserved this reflective moment, writing on their memory page, "The smells of good food cooking on holidays and special occasions, the remnants of his artwork looking back at us expressing his gentle kindness, the determination he had to learn to knit, and last but not least his calm bravery to face his journey (as our son described it). We loved Gil as if he were our own and will miss him dearly forever."

The final photo I encountered is of Gil and Jean, the creator of this memory book. The cropped photo showed the two of them smiling broadly into the camera lens. This photograph was showing its age, in a last flash of glowing yellows, before giving in to the natural, muted, fading process. Jean wrote, "His biting sense of humor and his knack to tell it like it is. Gil was a true gem. I know he's in his beautiful place watching over us, laughing with us."

As I thumbed through the book, I noticed for the first time all the different styles of handwriting. Sometimes more than one contribution crowded the page. Three pages were crisply typewritten. There were quotations, and there was poetry, both borrowed and original. Some pages were adorned with drawings. One page had three preprinted graphics gaily colored in by an adult, as if by a delighted child. Another page was stamped with multi-colored rubber stamps in the images of hearts, starbursts, and teddy bears holding hands.

I found this intimate collection a testimony, not only to Gil and his effect on others but also to our life together, and to my caregiving.

Many words describing Gil repeated throughout. Poignant phrases jumped out at me from the pages: "A dignity..." "Charming and warm..." "A heart so full of love and peace..." "Sweet, kind, and gentle..." "Always had a smile..." "Creativity flowed..." "Warmth and humor..." "How he finally found peace in his life..." "Full of courage..." "Gentle soul..." "Uncanny ability to lure in animals..." "Unconditional love and compassion..." "Easygoing manner..." "A true friend..." "Thought more of others than himself..." "Warm smile..." "Sexy moustache..." "Disarmingly honest and sometimes brutally frank..."

Recorded observations of our life together comforted me: "Gil and Andrew taught me to receive, to accept love and help." "Andy had given him stability, love, and a family he never quite had." "His love for Andy..." "Andrew faithfully and lovingly by his side..." "I hardly ever saw Gil without Andrew being somewhere nearby, protective, caring, loving, faithful, and patient." "Two individuals, but in my mind, one person..." "The bond that Andrew and he shared..." "The brightness in Gil's eyes whenever he spoke of Andy..." "It has been a privilege to witness the miracle of two human beings sharing each other's light and glowing so much more brightly; then sharing the radiance with the rest of us." "Whenever we see a sunrise we will reflect upon its beauty and remember Gil and Andrew."

There was also recognition of my caregiving as stated in one particular passage: "The calm saturated the room, a rich contentment in simply knowing Andrew was there; who has remained so strong and full of encouragement."

As I closed the "Memories of Gil" book for that day, I saw two phrases that reinforced the power, and the continuing importance, of the wisdom within its covers:

"May your memories stay with you always."

"Gil has gone home."

Acknowledgment and Thanks

For encouragement, for first readings, for providing a spiritually and emotionally supportive home, for promotion of my work in daily conversations, for love, and for partnership – Lev Baesh.

For suggesting I read Julia Cameron's *The Artist's Way* as a guide to start clearing my mind of all the stories I had been holding on to, stories I was fearful of forgetting – Jane Lesley.

For bringing me into the Molasses Pond writing sanctuary, for careful reading, for nurturing, and for writing support – Martha Barron Barrett and Susan Wheeler.

For the intimate monthly writers' group; fellow writers and wonderful friends experiencing the conception and completion of my manuscript. For spending countless Tuesday evenings critiquing my endless stories on caregiving and death – Rosemary A. Zurawel and Karen Towne.

For friends who believed in me and read and re-read many evolving drafts – Rabbi Ruth Alpers, Elizabeth Goldman, Kathy Gunst, Meg Kerr, and Kathy Bloomfield. For preparing us and assisting with Gil's peaceful journey – the volunteers and staff of Strafford Hospice Care/Seacoast Hospice, especially Angela Raney and Marjorie Edmunds.

For "re-discovering" my manuscript, and believing in it enough to help bring it to the world – Marilyn Traugott.

For making this the best caregiving book and learning tool that it could be – Karla Wheeler, Kelly Brachle, Traceé Young, Cayla Stanley and the staff at Quality of Life Publishing Company. For lending her editing skills – Carole Greene. And to Mark May, for designing such a meaningful cover.

For those readers to whose lives I hope to offer some caregiving inspiration and guidance, I am grateful that you shared with me the life journeys chronicled in this book.

And for ultimately giving me the gift to write, orchestrating all these cosmic connections, living all these stories with me during our brief time together and continuing after death, and guiding me to become an "End-of-Life Coach" – my eternal soulmate, Gil Victor Ornelas.

Appendices:
End-of-Life Coaching Excerises

For the following exercises, I encourage you to copy down the questions and your answers on a sheet of paper, or in a journal. Writing is a therapeutic activity that helps release emotions and organize thoughts. Many of these exercises have been adapted from the End-of-Life Nursing Education Consortium curriculum.

The End-of-Life Nursing Education Consortium (ELNEC) Project is a national end-of-life educational program administered by City of Hope National Medical Center (COH) and the American Association of Colleges of Nursing (AACN) designed to enhance palliative care in nursing. The ELNEC Project was originally funded by a grant from the Robert Wood Johnson Foundation with additional support from funding organizations (the National Cancer Institute, Aetna Foundation, Archstone Foundation, and California HealthCare Foundation). Materials are copyrighted by COH and AACN and are used with permission. Further information about the ELNEC Project can be found at **www.aacn.nche.edu/ELNEC**.

Appendix A:

End-of-Life Coaching Exercise
TWO QUESTIONS

1. Please ponder and record the answers to these two questions:

- *What apprehensions do you have about taking care of someone who is dying?*

- *What do you fear most about your own death?*

———————

Appendix B:

End-of-Life Coaching Exercise
PERSONAL LOSS INVENTORY

1. On a fresh sheet of paper, create a grid of five columns and five rows. Label the tops of each column with the following headings:

   My Five Favorite Possessions
   My Five Favorite Activities
   Five Essential Parts of My Body
   Five Important Values
   Five People I Love

2. Now imagine you have a terminal illness, with six months or less to live. If you had to give up one of these items, what would it be? Cross it out on the chart. Continue crossing out items in order of things you'd next be willing to give up, until everything is crossed out.

People living with a terminal illness face multiple losses as the disease progresses. Oftentimes, we do not have the choice of the order of what is being lost.

3. Write down and answer the following questions:

- *What did you cross out first?*

- *What did you cross out last?*

- *What emotions did you feel during this exercise?*

Appendix C:

End-of-Life Coaching Exercise
LIFELINE GRAPH

1. In your journal, draw a line that best represents your life, starting with birth and ending with death. Along the line, you will want to enter your birth date, present age, estimated age at death, milestones/lifecycle events that you have experienced, and those you expect to happen before you die. Be as creative as you wish.

2. Once you finish your line, take a look at what you have accomplished and what you have listed as unmet goals. Write down how this makes you feel.

Appendix D:

End-of-Life Coaching Exercise
YOUR FAMILY

1. Draw a picture of your family, considering both family of origin and family of choice. Be as creative as you can. If you are

not artistic, consider using various geometrical shapes and considering how the shapes may or may not interact. Identify each person in each shape.

2. Now look at your creation. Elisabeth Kübler-Ross identified five stages of coping as: Denial, Anger, Bargaining, Depression, and Acceptance. What stages are the identified family members in your picture currently experiencing regarding the anticipated loss of someone you love? What are your thoughts on these different stages you identified, stages that everyone may find themselves in?

Appendix E:
End-of-Life Coaching Exercise
PHILOSOPHY OF DEATH

1. What is your personal philosophy of death? Do you believe in an afterlife? Will death be a wall or a door for you? Journal your personal reflections of these questions, and elaborate on them, if you wish.

2. Do you feel comfortable sharing this personal philosophy of death with someone you love? If so, share. You may both find out more about yourself and the other person.

Appendix F:

End-of-Life Coaching Exercise
BEING PRESENT/LISTENING

1. Please do this exercise with another person. Find a comfortable setting, get a timer, and take turns being the "Speaker" and the "Listener."

- *The first Speaker"will describe a significant loss (person, object, activity) for five minutes. The Listener will listen in silence during those five minutes.*

- *Change roles. The Speaker becomes the Listener and the Listener becomes the Speaker for five minutes.*

2. After you are done taking turns being Speaker and Listener, write down the answers to the following questions for when you were the Speaker:

- *How did it feel to describe your loss?*

- *In what ways did the listener respond to you?*

3. Now answer these questions for when you were the Listener:

- *Was it difficult for you to listen in silence for five minutes?*

- *Does five minutes seem to be too short or too long a time period?*

4. What did you learn about yourself and about being present and listening from doing this exercise? Write your thoughts down in your journal.

We may feel uncomfortable spending time with someone who is dying, not knowing what to say. However, one of the greatest gifts that we can offer someone who is dying is our presence and listening.

———◦◦◦———

Appendix G:

End-of-Life Coaching Exercise
CULTURAL CONSIDERATIONS

1. Do you have cultural/religious/spiritual customs and rituals? If so, what are they? List them in your journal.

2. Which of the customs and rituals you listed do you feel need to be observed in your dying experience?

———◦◦◦———

Appendix H:

End-of-Life Coaching Exercise
OBITUARIES AND MEMORIAL SERVICES

1. Regardless of where you are in the caregiving trajectory, I would encourage you to plan to visit your local funeral home and speak with a funeral director to learn about pre-planning a funeral for you or someone you love.

2. Next, I would like you to read some obituaries from your local newspaper. Also read obituaries that appear in the *New York Times*. Compare and contrast what you find. Once you have become familiar with the formula of an obituary, choose a col-

ored sheet of paper and write your own obituary as you would like to see it printed in the newspaper.

How did you feel after completing this exercise? Write your feelings down.

3. Now take another sheet of a different colored paper. Title this sheet, "My Memorial/Celebration of Life Service." Describe who will be present, where the service will be held, and what readings and music will be used. What other details will be important to you on this day?

How did you feel after describing this future event?

4. I would encourage you to share these two documents with someone you love, if you are comfortable doing so. Alternatively, you may choose to put these away some place safe to reflect upon, to have this discussion at a later time.

Appendix I:
End-of-Life Coaching Exercise
REGRETS

1. Do you currently have any regrets for life goals that you have not met? If so, list your personal "What Ifs" and "If Onlys" in your journal.

2. Which of the listed "What Ifs" and "If Onlys" can you have the hope of achieving? Can you identify a date that you might be

able to meet this goal?

Even though someone may be facing a life-limiting illness, there should always be the hope for something: the hope to attend an upcoming family wedding; the hope to see the ocean or mountains one more time; the hope to have a peaceful, painless death.

Appendix J:
End-of-Life Coaching Exercise
RECONCILIATION

According to Dr. Ira Byock's book, *The Four Things That Matter Most,* the four things are: "Please forgive me," "I forgive you," "Thank you," and "I love you." Answer the following questions in your journal:

- *Is there someone in your life that you need to ask forgiveness? Who and why?*

- *Is there someone in your life that you need to forgive? Who and why?*

- *Is there someone in your life that you need to thank? Who and why?*

- *Is there someone in your life that you need to tell that you love? Who would that be?*

If you answered "yes" to any of these four things that matter most, please consider doing so today.

Appendix K:

End-of-Life Coaching Exercise

BECOME A DEATH AND DYING ADVOCATE

1. Lastly, I would encourage you to contact your local hospice organization and investigate what it takes to become a hospice volunteer; and I challenge you to make the commitment to become one. You may find that it will enrich your life in many ways.

2. Search for a local hospice through the website of the National Hospice and Palliative Care Organization, **www.nhpco.org**.

3. In your journal, write the name(s) and contact information of your local hospice organization.

If you need to learn more about the caregiving experience, the National Hospice and Palliative Care Organization website's Caring Connections section is an excellent resource. Visit **www.caringinfo.org**.

One goal of this book has been to start you on a personal journey of taking death "out of the closet." The more we talk about death amongst ourselves, the more it will shift from the institutionalized and medical event that it has become to the more intimate human experience that it can be.

Author Biography

Born 1954 in Portland, Maine, C. Andrew Martin gravitated toward his passions: writing, gardening, knitting, and generating hospice awareness. As a volunteer member of Seacoast Hospice's Speakers' Bureau, Andrew frequently read selections from this book, as it was evolving, to hospice training groups.

Preparation for writing this book includes his life experience as a caregiver for his partner Gil V. Ornelas; several writing workshops at the University of New Hampshire; attending the Molasses Pond Writers' Conferences at the request of its organizers (both published authors), Martha Barron Barrett and Susan Wheeler; and a self-formed writers' group that emerged from the Molasses Pond Conference.

Andrew has a passion for both hospice education and quality care. He began his hospice association in 1993, as a volunteer for Strafford Hospice Care, Rollinsford, New Hampshire, which later merged with Seacoast Hospice and is now Beacon Hospice, Inc.

Since writing this memoir, Andrew has become a Registered Nurse, focusing in hospice care, education, and quality. Currently employed by Beacon Hospice, Inc., Andrew is a Certified Hospice and Palliative Nurse who previously worked for Seacoast Hospice (2001-2008) in the roles of RN Case Manager, Intake and Clinical Support RN, and lastly on their management team as Education and Quality Assurance Performance Improvement (QAPI) Coordinator. He was instrumental in achieving recognition of a 2007 OCS Vision Award to Seacoast Hospice for exceptional efforts in strategic initiatives that improve quality of care and organizational excellence.

Andrew has achieved Level II Designee of the National Hospice and Palliative Care Organization's Hospice Manager Development Program (2007). He is also an approved educator by both the End-of-Life Nursing Education Consortium (ELNEC) Training Program (2006) and the Hospice and Palliative Nurse Association Clinical Review Trainer Program (2007). As Adjunct Faculty at the University of New Hampshire (2007-2008), Boston College (2010), and Saint Joseph's College of Maine (2010), Andrew taught the Death & Dying and Palliative Practicum courses to the next generation of healthcare professionals.

Hospice industry networking is important to Andrew. He has been the volunteer mentor (2005-2007) for the New Hampshire Hospice and Palliative Care Organization's initiative to successfully increase statewide participation in the NHPCO National Data Set (NDS).

His professional affiliations are with the Hospice and Palliative Care Federation of Massachusetts; Hospice and Palliative Nurses Association; Massachusetts Nurses Association; National Hospice and Palliative Care Organization; New Hampshire Hospice and Palliative Care Organization; New Hampshire Nurses Association; Oncology Nurses Society; Reform Jewish Nurses Network; Seacoast Oncology Nurses; and Sigma Theta Tau Iota Chapter.

In his downtime, Andrew enjoys bicycling, snowshoeing, the meditation of knitting, and spending time with his loving and supportive partner, Rabbi Lev Baesh, and their two Boston Terriers, Nefesh and Emet.

* * *

To order *Reflections of a Loving Partner: Caregiving at the End of Life* and other gentle grief support publications:

Bookstores: Available wherever books are sold

Online: www.QoLpublishing.com

Email: books@QoLpublishing.com

Phone: Call during regular business hours Eastern Time.
Toll free in the U.S. and Canada:
1-877-513-0099 or call 1-239-513-9907

Fax: **1-239-513-0088**

Mail: Quality of Life Publishing Co.
P.O. Box 112050
Naples, FL 34108-1929